AGING
SAFELY,
WISELY,
and
WELL

AGING SAFELY, WISELY, *and* WELL

A MOVEMENT AND MINDSET GUIDE *for* OLDER ADULTS

C. VICKI GOLD, PT, MA

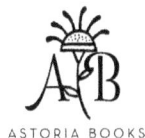

ASTORIA BOOKS

Published 2024
Printed in the United States of America
Paperback ISBN: 978-1-7364605-7-3
Library of Congress Control Number: 2024920224

Astoria Books
Seattle, WA
info@astoriabooks.com

Editing and book design by Stacey Aaronson, www.thebookdoctorisin.com
Illustrations by Lily Padula (pages 26, 37, 48–51, 83, 95, 110, 114, and 142), www.lilypadula.com

The information in this book is designed to help the reader make informed decisions about his/her health. It is not intended as a medical prescription or to replace the advice of the reader's own physician or other medical professional. It is not intended to replace any medical treatment offered by the reader's own doctors. Every reader should consult a medical professional in matters relating to health, especially if you have preexisting medical conditions. The author(s) and publisher do not accept responsibility for any adverse effects individuals may claim to experience, whether directly or indirectly, from the information contained in this book. The names and identifying characteristics of patients have been changed to protect their privacy.

This book is dedicated to all individuals who have overcome challenges of any kind in their lives and who aim to transform the ways they move through life, striving to make the world a better place for themselves and others.

and

To my loving and devoted husband, Tom Carbone,
who provided the support and solid foundation
that has allowed me to fly,
forever and ever.

Table of Contents

Introduction

I t's no secret that we are all aging. The question is: What can we do to age as safely and independently as possible? Even if you've stayed fit and active most or all of your life, it's possible that fear has crept in at one time or another about how you will function both mentally and physically in your later years. No one wants to imagine living with limited mobility, or having to give up work or hobbies they love, or not being able to have fun with their grandchildren—or worse, being dependent on others for their day-to-day care because of a fall or deteriorating health.

This is why I wrote this book: to show you steps you can take to be functionally fit—and better able to manage stress—for the rest of your life. You read that right! *For the rest of your life.* I'm not talking about becoming a bodybuilder or going to a gym five days a week or adding strenuous exercise sessions into your daily routine. I'm talking about simple things, such as learning correct bending and lifting techniques that can help you prevent unwanted back pain and injuries; using conscious breathing to reduce stress and combat anxiety; applying simple movement techniques that can foster the strength, flexibility, balance, and endurance you need to perform your everyday activities, whether at home or on the job.

Look, I get it. There are countless books, articles, websites, and professional experts with knowledge and ideas about how to age well, and many are excellent. Some are even referenced in the "My Favorite Things" section of this book. So, you're probably asking, "Why do we need another 'expert' book?"

and "Why is this book any different from the scores of available resources that offer valuable information on healthful aging, staying fit, aging in place, etc.?"

As a physical therapist for over fifty years, and having recently turned eighty at the time of this publication, I've had the advantage of decades of cultivating the knowledge and skills I'm going to share with you (and yes, that's a current photo of me on the cover!). Maybe these modalities, tips, and tricks won't be new to you; this is often the case when I've presented my work at conferences. However, in my experience, people often learn things of value, but they never actually make them part of their daily lives. What's more, many healthcare workers and professionals don't practice what they are taught in school—so not only do they fall prey to back pain, injuries, and declining health, but they are also less effective at helping their patients avoid suffering these setbacks.

In the mid-1980s, at a private studio in New York City, I had an opportunity to conduct a class for people with medical or physical conditions who felt unsafe or uncomfortable in a traditional gym setting. I called the class Thera-Fitness (after all, I was a physical *therapist* conducting a *fitness* class). From the beginning, my intention was to give class participants a foundation for safe, effective movement and function, not for "exercising," per se, but for performing everyday activities more safely and effectively. Ultimately, Thera-Fitness was incorporated with the mission statement "to inspire, empower, and educate people toward the goal of optimum health and fitness."

As I led these Thera-Fitness classes, I came to develop what became "The ABC Mind-Body System"—a simple mnemonic for the core of achieving better overall physical function: **Alignment**, **Breathing**, and **Centering**. Experience has shown that these three components can impact not only how you look, feel, and function, but also help you be mentally calmer, be better at managing or at least minimizing stress, and coping more effectively with life's responsibilities and challenges. These ABCs became the basis for this book, along with additional strategies and techniques that can help you achieve the above goals, all of which you'll find in the following pages.

I realize that at this point, you may be wondering if this book is for you, with concerns and questions such as:

* My joints are getting stiffer and achier as I age. Will this book help me alleviate that?

* I'm feeling weaker and less agile with each passing year. Will I learn how to increase my strength and flexibility?

* I'm afraid of falling. Will you teach me ways to improve my balance?

* I wish I had more energy for doing the things I love. Will the activities in this book help with that?

* I'm worried about being able to "age in place." Will I learn ways to remain physically independent?

* I'm a younger adult and not ready to think about aging. Should I read this book?

* I've always heard you can't teach an old dog new tricks. Will this book have value for me if I'm already in my 80s or 90s?

* I'm frail and can't exercise anymore. Will Thera-Fitness and these ABCs apply to me?

* I have chronic obstructive pulmonary disease (COPD). Will your mind-body approach work for me in my condition?

* I don't have a medical or physical condition. I just want to look and feel as good as I can. Will the guidance in this book help me achieve that?

No matter which of these may apply to you—even if you doubt that you can improve the quality of your mobility, flexibility, and balance—the answer to all of these questions is a resounding YES. I can tell you from years of experience that the techniques I lay out for you in this book have the power to prevent and even reverse some of the challenges we "older adults" face, such as joint pain and stiffness, loss of functional muscle strength, and decreased balance with its resultant "fear of falling." And yes, for you younger adults, it's now that you can start preventing many of the challenges of old age.

For those of you hoping to "age in place," you probably have an even stronger motivation to stay mentally and physically fit. The information and skill training that follows will be especially valuable in helping you achieve that goal—and "practicing your ABCs" will be an easy way to remember and apply the beneficial skills you'll be learning here!

For those who hate exercise or believe you can't do it, I want to emphasize that Thera-Fitness is *not* an "exercise" program. It is a collection of mental strategies and movement skills that most people can do; even if you can only manage the conscious Breathing activity in my ABC program to begin with, you will benefit tremendously. Ideally, you will eventually be able to integrate each of the five ABC system elements into your everyday life, along with the additional mind-body skills presented in this book. Physically, you will find yourself standing taller, breathing more deeply, and feeling stronger, more confident, and fit for a life of functional independence. Mentally, you may be surprised at how much calmer and better able to handle potentially stressful situations you are.

So, whether you have a physically and mentally active life or a quieter lifestyle, I want to encourage you that there is still plenty you can do to maximize your mobility, functional independence, and even energy! Just wait until we discuss neuroplasticity in Chapter 1—you'll be impressed and maybe even blown away by the fact that you are truly *never* too old or too frail to gain benefits from making even the slightest change in your routine.

The work we will do together in this book is based on my professional education in traditional medicine—which included anatomy, kinesiology, psychology, and ergonomics—and is adapted from my experience with many mind-body trainings, which have included yoga, Pilates, and tai chi, as well as Alexander and Feldenkrais Techniques, all of which stimulate mental and physical fitness and well-being. (You can read more about these in the Glossary.) Further, my work with psychologists, and seminars by Landmark Worldwide, have contributed to the strategies presented in this book for managing stress, developing a positive mindset, and increasing productivity.

I was also aided in the writing of this book by multiple contributors, each of whom is highly experienced and passionate about their work. I am grateful for their commitment and willingness to deepen your appreciation of what it takes to age as safely, wisely, and well as you can.

As you work your way through this book, I encourage you to try out each of the different strategies and techniques that are presented. Some may feel a little awkward, strange, or even funny at first, and some may be a bit challenging. But don't be tempted to give up too quickly. Try them with an attitude of play and exploration. Just like when you go shopping for clothes, some will fit better than others, and some will make you feel better than others. Still others will take time to adapt to. But if you keep your goals in mind—like maintaining or enhancing your strength and flexibility, improving your balance, having more energy for doing the things you love, being able to "age in place," etc.— you will likely find out just how capable and full of potential you truly are!

To help you begin to experience the transformation we are talking about, we'll first explore a few powerful keys that are foundational to aiding you in identifying and reaching your goals.

Chapter 1

Setting Yourself Up for Successful Transformation: The Power of Neuroplasticity, Mindfulness, and Visualization

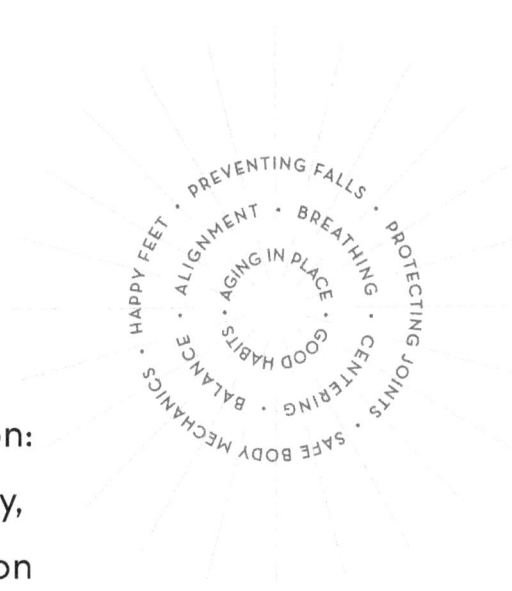

You're no doubt aware of the mind-body connection, and perhaps that awareness is a big part of your life already. Volumes have been written about it, and proof of it abounds—from how thoughts affect your physical body, to how many athletes visualize their performance to perfect it, to changing our own capabilities simply by how we speak to ourselves (more on that in Chapter 5), and so much more!

For me, my appreciation of the mind-body relationship was developed over years of personal experiences and working with patients as a physical therapist—but the most dramatic personal experience came during a doubles tennis match in Brazil. I was fortunate to have an opportunity to live, work, and teach there in the mid 1970s, and I had been invited to play by people who were infinitely more expert at tennis than I was.

From the beginning of the match, I was completely intimidated. My missed returns were showing how inept I was, and I was becoming more nervous by the minute. Then, something happened. I suddenly remembered the breathing technique I had learned in a recent meditation class. I started using it and within minutes I was laser-focused on the shots coming my way. My routine now became *Breathe – Focus – Spot the ball – Return the ball.* As I repeated this process, I was soon playing like a pro. I can still sense the confusion among my teammates as my game turned on a dime. It was the first time I actually experienced the undeniable results of the mind-body connection at work!

In this chapter, I'm going to introduce you (or reintroduce you if you're already familiar with the following material) to how mindfulness and visualization are incredible tools as you strive to make positive and healthful changes in how your mind and body function. But before we do that, I want to touch briefly on how I've structured most of the topics in this book.

To make the guidance easy to follow, as well as to give you a deeper understanding of how and why to do each item, I will pose the following questions: "What is it?" "Why is it important?" and "How do you achieve it?" I also often ask, "When should you do it?" For most strategies and techniques, the answer will almost always be: whenever possible throughout your day! While this may seem redundant to see over and over again, I've found it's a helpful reminder when incorporating something new into your daily routine. This structure also supports the tagline of Thera-Fitness: "Transforming the ways you move through life," which is precisely what I aim to help you do throughout this book.

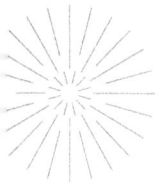

NEUROPLASTICITY

What Is It?

Neuroplasticity is the brain's capacity to continue growing and evolving in response to life experiences. As *plasticity* is the capacity to be shaped, molded, or altered, *neuroplasticity* is the ability for the brain to adapt or change over time by creating new neurons and building new networks.

Why Is It Important?

So few people realize we can transform our brain as we age—*if* we stimulate it. Once you know that the brain can continue to learn and grow throughout our lives, the sky is the limit for effecting positive changes—at all ages! This means it is possible to shift dysfunctional and unproductive patterns of thinking and behaving and to develop healthy, more constructive and positive mindsets, new memories, new skills, and new abilities.

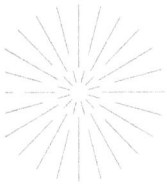

How Do You Achieve It?

There are endless ways to keep your brain elastic—take up a new hobby, learn another language, read up on subjects you're curious about, pick up a sport, take a class, do crossword puzzles, nurture a garden, play games, interact with children . . . the list goes on. Essentially, when you engage in any activity that forces the brain to think or contemplate new information or skills, or to see the world from a different perspective, you have the power to keep your brain in tip-top shape. An excellent video that debunks the attitude that you can't teach an old dog new tricks can be found here:

https://bit.ly/new-tricks-neuroplasticity

One of the most powerful ways to open up "windows of plasticity" in the brain is physical activity. Aerobic exercise, the kind that increases your heart rate and promotes enhanced oxygen use, boosts both heart and brain health by stimulating the release of the substance known as brain-derived neurotropic factor (BDNF). This element sets in motion the growth of new synaptic connections and bolsters the strength of signals transmitted from neuron to neuron. As these networks of neuronal correction are paved, mental and behavioral flexibility increase.

Stress is known to weaken expression of BDNF (one of many reasons to mitigate stress, which we'll address in the next chapter when we talk about breathing techniques). But studies show that walking an hour a day, five days a week boosts BDNF, which increases brain matter in the hippocampus, the seat of learning and memory. If you're not able to walk an hour a day, an alternative would be any activity—even one done sitting—that increases your heart rate and causes you to breathe more deeply.

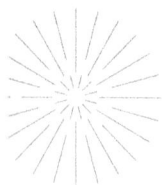

When Should You Do It?

Every day, as you think of it, find new and creative ways to stretch your mind and body's skills, even if they feel awkward in the beginning!

MINDFULNESS

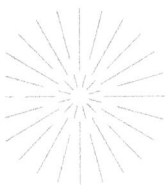

What Is It?

Often called "being in the moment," mindfulness is a state of mental peace and openness, wherein you hold subtle awareness of your internal and external environments. Deepak Chopra, in his book *12 Weeks to a Sharper You*, describes it as "the simple act of paying attention and noticing and being present in whatever you're doing."

Note here that mindfulness is distinct from *meditation*, which is a more formal practice. (There are many types of meditation, several of which are focused on specific goals—opening your heart, expanding your awareness, calming your mind, experiencing inner peace, connecting with a higher power, the list goes on. An abundance of books and resources exist for embarking on this practice, so we will not explore this topic here.) What's important for you to know is that while meditation is a wonderful practice and I highly recommend it, it is not necessary for being "mindful."

Why Is It Important?

When you are actively mindful, you notice the world around you, as well as your thoughts, feelings, behaviors, movements, and effects you have on others. Rather than merely jumping from one task to the next, or being absorbed in yourself alone, mindfulness allows you to fully experience all aspects of life as a human being—and to engage with others in a positive way. In addition, it develops crucial awareness of both our external and internal environments that can keep you safe, such as:

* Recognizing hazards in your *external* environment, helping you avoid costly falls, accidents, and mistakes.

* Being aware of *internal* sensations, which can alert you to signs that something is not right and may need attention, like tightness in your chest or an ache in your stomach.

* Urging you to consciously focus and stop multitasking, a known risk for accidents, injuries, and mistakes. (How often have you had an accident or injury when your mind was thinking one thing, but your body was doing something else? We'll learn the Stop–Act–Stop strategy for managing all those items on your to-do list later in this book.)

Yet another benefit of the sensations and awarenesses you gain with mindfulness is that it may help you decide to develop or change certain **habits**. Of course we have many that are useful and give order to our lives, like brushing our teeth morning and night, putting our keys in the same place at home, or taking an afternoon walk. These habits contribute to our health and well-being, and we generally have positive attitudes about them, especially when we understand their purpose and value. But what about habits of thought and physical action that are less constructive? Those that interfere with our health, our ability to achieve our goals, or to merely function well on a daily basis, such as smoking, overeating, drinking alcohol, sitting for long periods, etc.?

Being mindful allows you to thoughtfully reflect on some of your habits and ask: Which ones are beneficial to my health, life, and well-being? Which ones are harmful or even destructive? Which leads to: Which habits do I want to keep because they make me feel good and are good for me? Which ones am I better off losing? The chapters that follow will likely alert you to both, and hopefully encourage you toward the more healthful ones.

Finally, mindfulness will serve you well as you start integrating "The ABC Mind-Body System" into your everyday life. You'll want to ask yourself questions like:

* How do the recommended activities feel?
* Do they help me move more freely?
* Do they make me stand taller?
* Am I breathing more freely and deeply?
* Am I reducing stress?
* Am I functioning more safely and efficiently?

As you assess these questions, you'll find yourself actively involved in the activity with all of your senses, in the present moment, gently bringing yourself back to the task at hand instead of allowing your mind to wander. As you do this, you will begin to "transform the ways you move through life."

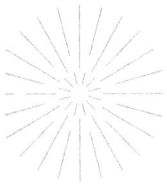

How Do You Achieve It?

My friend Matt Jeffs, a physical therapist who teaches mindfulness, uses a great analogy for what it takes to develop the practice. He says to consider the untrained mind to be like a puppy that's being taught to "sit." Just like a puppy, your mind needs constant cuing and positive reinforcement (yelling and punishment are not effective for animals *or* humans, so please be kind to yourself and don't resort to these negative tactics!). And, just like it is natural for a puppy to run off when you're trying to train it, it is natural for your mind to wander off as you practice becoming more mindful. So "invite it back" and eventually, the "puppy" will come when you call it.

Another step in mindfulness training is to slow down (we'll explore the art and benefits of this in Chapter 3) and allow the integration of body awareness and breathing, meaning sensing your mind and body working together.

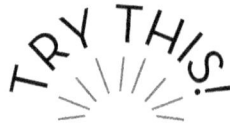

TRY THIS!

Get into a comfortable, supported position—lying or sitting, it doesn't matter.

Close your eyes and turn your attention to your breathing. What do you notice?

- Is your breathing fast or slow?

- Is it high in your chest or does the air go down toward your belly?

- Are you relaxed, or are you noticing areas of pain or tension?

Try to avoid judging what you are doing or how you are feeling. Just notice. This is a basic exercise in mindfulness.

(We'll talk more about "conscious breathing" in the next chapter, but for now, simply pay attention—or "tune in"—to how your body feels.)

THE 3-4-4-3 TECHNIQUE

I learned this technique from Judith Grant, RN, at Pathways to Health in New York.

1. Find a quiet place and get seated or positioned comfortably.

2. Close your eyes as you become mindful of your breathing.

3. Take 3 slow breaths, in through your nose, out through your nose (or mouth, if that's more comfortable).

4. While taking the next 4 breaths, say or think the word "deeper" with each one.

5. During the next 4 breaths, think of a word that brings you inner calm. (My usual word is "peace," but it could be "love," "joy," "harmony," or any single word that makes you feel light, positive, and just plain good.)

6. Your next 3 breaths will bring you back to reality, hopefully in a calm and relaxed state.

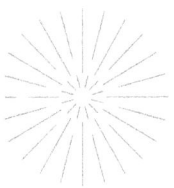

When Should You Do It?

The beauty of mindfulness is that you can practice it anytime, anywhere, and with anyone by being fully engaged in the here and now. Many people go about their daily lives with their minds wandering from the activity they are participating in to other thoughts, desires, fears, or wishes—but all it takes is "calling the puppy back" to anchor you in the present moment.

VISUALIZATION

What Is It?

Visualization, also called imagery, is where you use your imagination to picture yourself in a specific situation, or performing a certain task or skill.

Why Is It Important?

Science has shown that the body doesn't actually know the difference between real and imagined situations. This is why watching an intense movie, even though you're not in the suspenseful or violent scene yourself, creates bodily reactions that mimic fight or flight—your body's innate response to saving you from a perceived threat. In this same vein, picturing yourself in a calm environment, such as next to a waterfall, on a quiet beach, or in a mountain retreat, lowers cortisol levels in the body, which in turn lowers stress.

Taking visualization to another level, you can use it to create a more positive mindset, or to mentally practice a task or skill. Elite athletes train this way, and you can do it too—for any task or skill you wish to achieve or improve. To illustrate how the brain works when imagery is engaged, and how athletes use it to their advantage, I highly recommend the excellent video below:

https://bit.ly/5-visualization-techniques

Visualization is a powerful tool to use for your transformation, and I am confident you'll find it empowering.

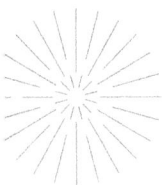

How Do You Achieve It?

What follows are two excellent activities for practicing visualization.

Imagine yourself in a situation where you feel loved, supported, happy, etc. Notice how your body feels. Are you sensing your muscles relaxing? Are you breathing more deeply? Do you have a sense of inner peace? Notice how nothing has changed in your external world, yet your internal world transformed (there's that word again!).

....

Visualize a physical skill you want to improve or develop. It could be anything from rising easily from a sitting position to learning a sport. To take a simple example, let's say you'd like to walk with more grace and ease.

Imagine you are standing tall, breathing deeply, and striding with long steps. Your hips shift easily over each leg as your feet progress in a smooth heel-to-toe action. (You might liken this to walking on a sandy beach with your feet fully engaged in moving forward in the soft sand.) This aliveness and mobility in your feet is what you want to "wake up" in the brain.

As you picture doing this, your body is actually learning and practicing that skill, even if you are merely imagining it. Now, when you begin to walk in real time, you have a much better chance of achieving the goal of a more balanced and youthful gait.

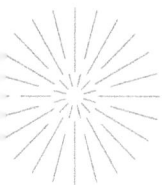

When Should You Do It?

Set aside "me" time to develop your ability to visualize changes you'd like to see in yourself, or even in the world around you. The great news is, you need zero tools except for your own imagination to practice visualization.

A great way to make it part of your routine is to develop a trigger. For example, if you lapse into any negative thinking or begin to affirm certain unfavorable conditions ("I'll never be able to do this," "My body aches," "This weather is so depressing" . . . you get the idea), let it be a wakeup call to stop and visualize something positive. You may have many tasks, skills, or even heightened well-being you'd like to accomplish, or you may have a single predominant goal. Whatever your circumstance, I recommend choosing one, visualizing the outcome you want to achieve, and starting to build those brain connections to make it become a reality.

With neuroplasticity, mindfulness, and visualization as tools in your transformation toolbox, let's move on to discovering how beneficial it can be to make the ABC Mind-Body System a transformative part of your daily life.

Chapter 2

Making The ABC Mind-Body System a Transformative Part of Your Daily Life

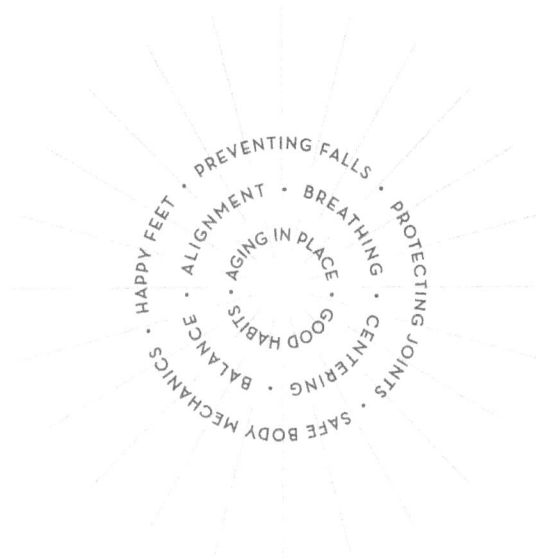

S ome years ago, I was the director of the Physical Therapist Assistant Program at LaGuardia Community College in New York. My students were tasked with learning a great deal of information before graduating, and one day a student came into my office highly distressed.

"How am I ever going to learn all this material?!" she cried.

"You're not," I calmly told her. "We're just planting seeds here. You're going to be watering them for the rest of your life."

To you, dear reader, I say the same: The ABC Mind-Body System will encourage you to plant seeds—seeds you will hopefully be inspired to continue watering for the rest of your life.

With those life-changing seeds in mind, let's dive into what The ABC Mind-Body System is all about!

A = ALIGNMENT

What Is It?

Simply stated, postural alignment is the position of your various body parts in relation to each other. Unfortunately, as many of us age, especially if we have not consciously managed our posture, changes happen. The diagram below is taken from the outstanding work of Sara Meeks, physical therapist, geriatric specialist, and yoga instructor.

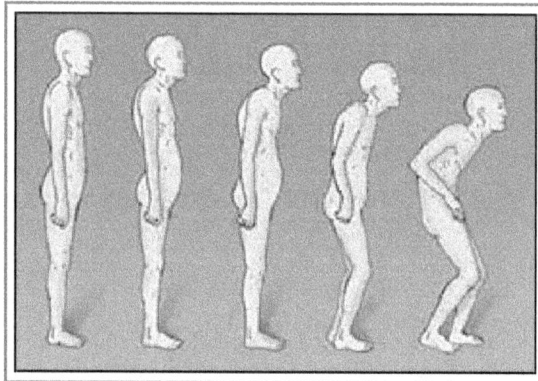

Why Is It Important?

There are both physical and mental reasons that good postural Alignment is beneficial:

* **Your body parts function through their fuller ranges of motion,** giving you improved freedom of movement. You'll see this when you try the activity on the next page.

* **Your internal organs have more room to function properly,** particularly your lungs, stomach, and intestines.

* **Your balance improves as your body segments line up.** Think about how stacked blocks won't fall if one is directly on top of the other. Now think of your body as a series of stacked blocks. As soon as one is out of alignment, especially the top one (your head), the risk of them falling is greater.

* **It promotes self-esteem.** For example, if you have low self-esteem, do you notice that your posture matches that feeling? In other words, do you carry yourself in a slouched manner? Or do you maybe avoid good posture because you relate it to appearing "snooty"? What if you simply pulled yourself upright—not in an exaggerated "snooty" way, but naturally. I dare you not to feel heightened self-esteem and confidence!

* **It improves mood, sense of well-being, and confidence.**

* **It enhances mental alertness.**

TRY THIS!

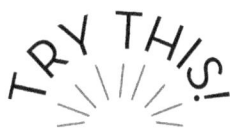

DEVELOPING POSTURAL AWARENESS

Look at your body in a full-length mirror. Take a moment to notice how you look and feel. Note the position of your head on your neck. Does it press forward? Can you tuck your chin and press your head back without looking up?

What about the position of your shoulders? Do they roll up and forward, compressing your chest? Can you press them down and back?

When you are standing, does your pelvis tip forward, causing your back to arch and your stomach to stick out? If so, can you tuck your pelvis under, causing your lower back to flatten instead?

This awareness will give you a sense of your postural alignment. Once you make the appropriate shifts, as seen below, it can make a notable difference in how you look, feel, and function.

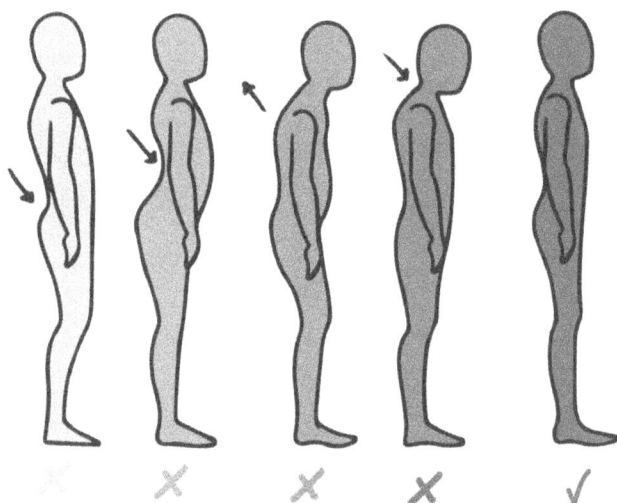

NOW THIS . . .

Still standing in front of the full-length mirror, look at your face.

Next, pull yourself up to your tallest posture. Without doing anything else, tell me you don't look better, and maybe even feel a little more confident!

FEEL THE DIFFERENCE!

1. Sit slouched with your pelvis slid forward in a straight-backed chair.

2. Raise one arm up as high as possible and close to your head. Notice how far it goes and how it feels.

3. Lower your arm back down.

4. Turn your head to one side. How far does it go? How does it feel?

....

1. Now, get a small cushion or towel-roll and place it behind the small of your back (lower arch, or lumbar spine) as you sit way back in this chair once again. If the chair has armrests, place your arms on those for support; if not, choose a chair seated at a desk, tabletop, etc., where you can rest your arms comfortably on top. Either way, your back should be as straight as possible.

2. Begin breathing in a slow, relaxed fashion. (More on a technique for this shortly, but for now, just breathe as slowly and relaxed as you can).

3. Now, repeat the arm-raising and head-turning movements you did when you were sitting slouched in the chair. Pay attention to any differences in how far you can do each move and whether it feels easier than the first time.

You should experience a marked difference. See what a small shift in posture can do?

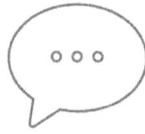

Mrs. S. arrived early for her physical therapy appointment with me. When I came out to greet her and prepare for our session, I noticed that she was seated, somewhat slouched, in the waiting room chair. I asked her to tell me the problem she was having.

She winced as she tried to lift her right arm, raising it only a few inches off her lap. "I can't lift it. It hurts."

My awareness of the benefits of postural alignment and conscious breathing kicked into action. "Let me help you get comfortable while you're waiting," I said. I assisted her in moving her hips back into the chair and placed a rolled towel at the small of her back. I then placed a pillow on her lap so she could rest her arms on it. Finally, I suggested that she focus on taking slow, relaxed breaths until our appointment time, which was in fifteen minutes.

When I returned to bring Mrs. S. in for her physical therapy treatment, I was curious how she felt. Once again, I asked her to raise her right arm. To both our amazement and joy, her arm went all the way up—and there was no wincing! I could have sent her home with nothing more than instructions on how to manage her posture!

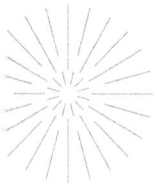

How Do You Achieve It?

As we discussed in Chapter 1, one of the best methods for achieving goals is the use of **visualization**, or **imagery.** In the same way that athletes regularly picture the result they hope to achieve in a meet, game, or competition, you can hold a set of mental pictures or images in your mind for any type of goal.

Because your body responds to images you create in the mind, the benefits can be mental as well as physical. It's an excellent tool toward achieving consistent postural alignment.

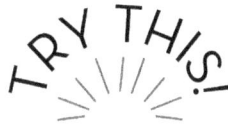

TRY THIS!

IMAGINING GOOD POSTURAL ALIGNMENT

Say out loud or to yourself: "**Lengthen – Open – Make space in your chest**."

Let's break these components down so they make sense.

The word **lengthen** tends to cause the "core" muscles to work. If you're not familiar with the core muscles, they are the deep muscles that surround your trunk, or torso—front, sides, back, top, and bottom. They support the spine and are necessary for attaining good postural alignment. (We will talk more about the core muscles and how to strengthen them in Chapter 6.) To attain a lengthened image in your mind, think of images that cause you to stand or sit with your best posture, such as, "I am a king/queen," or "I am tall, strong, and confident." As you do this, you get an opportunity to experiment and play with images and to also get a sense of how the mind and body affect each other.

The word **open** is to encourage your neck and shoulder muscles to relax when you straighten your posture. It is common to tighten those muscles when told to "stand up straight." But those muscles actually have nothing to do with helping you improve your posture, as they are not part of the core muscles that support the spine. To achieve a sense of openness, think of images or words that help you create a feeling of softness around your neck and shoulders. I like the image of a silk shirt draped loosely over a hanger. (Besides becoming more aware of your mind-body connection, you are utilizing the concept of "self-talk." More about that later.)

The phrase "**make room in your chest**" came from a woman in one of my classes. I tried it and found that it made my shoulders drop down and back even more, which made my chest expand more.

Now you try it!

1. Sit or stand with support, if needed, with or without your eyes closed.

2. Say aloud, or think the words, "**Lengthen - Open — Make space in your chest**." Notice as your body gets taller and straighter, your neck and shoulder muscles relax, your shoulders drop down and back, and your chest expands. I have also begun saying the phrase, "**Tuck your chin - Let the crown of your head rise toward the ceiling**," which many people find helpful as well.

REALIGNING YOUR HEAD AND NECK

Frequently, poor posture includes a "forward-head" position, as illustrated below.

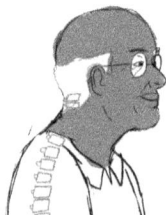

The way to correct this is to do a "chin tuck," also known as a chin retraction. This "pulling in" movement is standard for realigning your head on your trunk. If you're unsure how to accomplish this movement, the YouTube video below offers a good example of the technique. Just remember to align before you begin!

https://bit.ly/neck-retraction

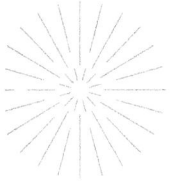

When Should You Do It?

Anytime you sit or stand, try to become aware of your posture. If it helps, ask yourself, *How am I standing?* each time you stand, and *How am I sitting?* each time you sit. After a while, you won't need the questions. Your postural alignment will become automatic—it just takes consistent reminders. And once you're aligned, you'll hopefully feel so much better that you won't want to slouch anymore!

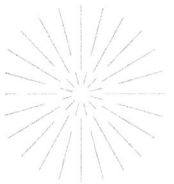

Tips to Achieve Improved Postural Alignment

Select seating that has the following considerations:

a.   It is well-suited to your size, allowing your back, feet, and even your arms to be supported. You want to have a hand's width of space between the front of the seat of the chair to the back of your knees, to avoid pressure behind your knees, and you want to be able to slide your hand between the underside of your thigh and the seat of the chair to avoid pressure there. Short people (like me!) often need a footstool and back cushion, since many chairs are too deep or high for us. Again, you want to avoid having pressure behind or under your knees.

Note: If you are taller than average, you may need custom furniture to achieve this.

b. Sit at a desk or table so your arms can be supported. That will create less of a downward pull on your spine and make sitting straight easier.

c. If you find you require special support, adaptive seating may be needed.

Again, this is a good time to use "Lengthen-Open" or other mental imagery (visualization), like picturing a thread coming from the top of your head and pulling it upward so that your spine is maximally lengthened.

Avoid leaning on only one armrest in a way that your body tilts to one side. This promotes poor alignment and undue pressure on the spine.

Whenever sitting in a chair, try to have your feet, arms, and back well supported. Use cushions, back supports, a foot stool, etc., to achieve the greatest comfort and postural alignment. Adjustable desks and chairs are particularly helpful for this.

B = BREATHING

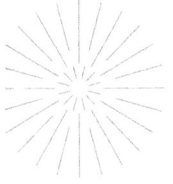

What Is It?

It may seem silly to define breathing when it's something we do thousands of times a day, mostly without thinking about it. But it's precisely because of the mindless way most of us breathe, and how little we tend to think about what oxygen does for the body (besides keeping us alive!) that we offer more discussion.

Put simply, plants and trees produce oxygen, and when we take that oxygen in through our nose or mouth, it fuels the body and provides energy for the cells that give us life. In turn, the carbon dioxide (CO_2) we exhale provides life to the plants and trees around us. It's a beautiful dance between humans and nature where each one is vital and sustains the other. (It is estimated that one tree can produce enough oxygen for ten people to breathe for a year!)

For two excellent demonstrations, I recommend watching the following brief videos:

https://tinyurl.com/scotland-breathing-animation
https://tinyurl.com/lung-anatomy-animation

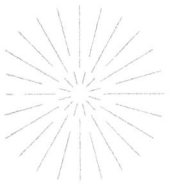

Why Is It Important?

Although breathing is mostly an automatic activity, it's critical to develop awareness of *how* you are breathing—or rather, making breathing *conscious*. When you do, you'll be amazed at what an incredible tool it is to increase your physical and mental well-being.

1. **Increased Lung Capacity.** When you *consciously* breathe, you make the best use of your lungs and breathing muscles, which then increases your respiratory (lung) capacity. What results is enhanced energy and endurance.

2. **Stress Reduction and Increased Calmness.** *Conscious* breathing, even in short sessions during the day, can put you into a state of calm. Have you ever noticed that when you're watching a suspenseful show or movie, or when you're trying to do something difficult, you hold your breath? Or, perhaps you find yourself breathing with short, shallow breaths? Either one sends an SOS to the vagus nerve, which can activate the fight-or-flight stress reaction without you even realizing it. (Read more about the vagus nerve in the Glossary on pages 193–94.) Though you may not feel stressed in the moment, your body is reacting negatively. Becoming aware of your altered breathing pattern, and initiating conscious breathing, is a way to keep the vagus nerve happy— and therefore your body happy. Bonus: you feel calmer and more relaxed too.

How Do You Achieve It?

Achieving conscious, diaphragmatic breathing is easy! All you have to do is become aware of your breathing rhythm and take control *consciously*. Here's how!

MASTERING DIAPHRAGMATIC BREATHING

The diaphragm is your primary muscle for breathing in (inhalation). If you find yourself using the muscles around your upper chest and neck to breathe in rather than using the diaphragm, which is in the upper abdomen, the following exercise will be of tremendous help to you. Also, diaphragmatic breathing helps you fill your lungs more completely, which becomes especially important if you're someone whose lung function is decreased or limited by a condition like chronic obstructive pulmonary disease (COPD) or emphysema.

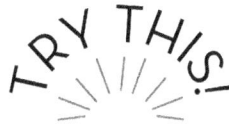

TRY THIS!

1. Sit or lie in a comfortable, supported position.

2. Close your eyes and turn your attention to your breathing. Without trying to change anything, notice if it is fast, slow, high in your chest, or down in your belly. What else do you notice? Are you breathing through your mouth or nose? The point is simply to come into awareness about your normal state of breathing.

3. Now, *consciously* slow the rate of your breaths. If you generally breathe through your mouth, **try to breathe through your nose** (see the next page for the importance of this). If your breath is high in your chest, strive to let your stomach expand as you breathe in.

4. Next, place your hands gently on your abdomen, just under your rib cage and slightly to the sides of your trunk. Make sure your chest is relaxed and your shoulders are down (not elevated in a shrugged-up position).

5. Now, imagine filling a balloon in your abdomen with air as you inhale. We call this "Balloon Breathing." Another image is inhaling your favorite fragrance (mine is lavender these days).

6. Become conscious of your abdomen expanding as you breathe in. (This is not meant to be an extreme "deep breath," which would force your chest to rise and your chest and neck muscles to tighten, but rather a gentle inhalation so you can feel the diaphragm working.)

7. Next, purse your lips, as if to whistle, as you prepare to exhale. You can also make a hissing sound between your teeth, like you'd hear from a leaky tire.

8. Time how long you can sustain pursed-lip or "leaky-tire" breathing. (Count to yourself or use the second hand of a clock or watch to time your endurance.)

9. Although you can exhale using either your nose or mouth, I encourage you to practice slow, prolonged exhalations through pursed lips. For the person with COPD, this helps stale or "residual" air, and possible secretions, be removed from the corners of your lungs, making more room for oxygenated air when you breathe in again.

WHY IT'S IMPORTANT TO BREATHE THROUGH YOUR NOSE

Breathing in through your nose allows air to be warmed, moistened, and filtered in a way that breathing in through the mouth does not. (If you are a "mouth breather," whether during waking or sleeping hours, or both, speak to your health or fitness professional about using "mouth tape" to retrain your breathing technique.) Also, air inhaled through the nose produces nitrous oxide, which aids in circulation.

FOR FUN!

Blow on a pinwheel or blow up balloons to provide great exercise for expiratory muscles and your ability to develop the prolonged exhalation I recommend.

Learn to prevent holding your breath when doing a strenuous activity by slowly counting out loud *before* you initiate the activity. This helps ensure that you don't hold your breath as you are exerting yourself.

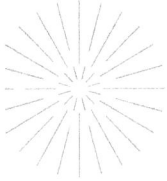

How Often Should You Practice These Breathing Techniques?

Every time you think of it! If you've never thought of conscious breathing before, a strategy could be to set a timer, maybe four or five times a day, as a reminder to practice these breathing techniques. Try to do at least 15 to 20 minutes during each session. You'll be amazed at how much calmer you feel, and you'll be doing your body an enormous favor by communicating to the vagus nerve that "all is well."

Once you are comfortable with conscious breathing, strive to do it at every opportunity. Some easy ways to do this are:

- If you watch a half-hour TV program, try to do *conscious breathing* during the entire show.

- If you listen to podcasts or audiobooks, make your listening time a *conscious-breathing* time as well.

- If you're stuck in traffic, be excited that the delay is actually triggering a time for *conscious breathing* (and bonus: it will reduce the stress you feel in traffic!).

- If you take naps, practice *conscious breathing* as you drift off.

- Make falling asleep at night a time to do *conscious breathing* (which also carries the benefit of sending you into dreamland in a relaxed state at the end of the day).

Depending on your life circumstances, look to find conscious, diaphragmatic breathing triggers throughout your day. Before you know it, you'll be consciously breathing without having to set timers to remind you because you'll notice how much better you feel in mind, body, and spirit when you do it regularly.

C = CENTERING

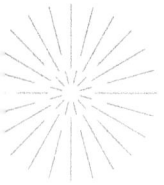

What Is It?

Within The ABC Mind-Body System, Centering has three meanings:

1. Allowing the mind and body to work together.
2. Moving from your "Center of Gravity" (COG).
3. Holding or lifting something or someone, or moving an object by keeping it close to your COG.

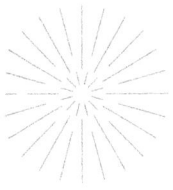

Why Is It Important?

1. **Mind and Body Working Together.** Have you ever had an accident or injury, or made a mistake because your mind was in one place, while your body was doing something else? I know I have! In this section, you'll learn a simple strategy for staying centered while performing tasks.

2. **Moving from Your "Center of Gravity" (COG).** For the average person, this is the area just below and behind your belly button when you are standing. (You see beautiful examples of people moving from their COG as they practice tai chi.) Learning to move from your COG improves your ability to balance and move more efficiently, and improved balance is a major factor to help you prevent falls.

3. **Holding Objects You Are Lifting or Moving Close to Your COG.** Have you ever tried to hold a bag of groceries, or a grandchild, out on extended arms? If so, you know how that puts a strain on your arms and back. Holding them close to your COG is not only biomechanically more efficient, but it reduces your risk of pain and injury, especially to your neck, back, and shoulders.

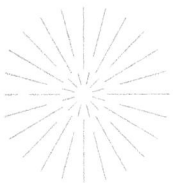

How Do You Achieve It?

1. My favorite strategy for keeping my **mind and body working together** is one I learned in a Landmark Worldwide seminar. I've changed it slightly and call it the "Start-Act-Stop" strategy. It is based on the premise that multitasking is *not* the most effective way to accomplish things safely and efficiently.

HERE'S HOW!

Start: This is the beginning of any project or task, no matter how big, small, or involved it may be. You will set your focus on this single task.

Act: This is when you are doing the particular activity. It could be as simple as washing a dish or talking on the phone, or as complex as taking on a large, involved project. It doesn't matter. What *does* matter is that you allow no distractions for the amount of time you're doing this task—no phone alerts, no interruptions to your call, no checking email, social media, etc.

Stop: This is when you reach the end of an activity—the dish is in the drainer, the phone conversation has ended, or you've reached a stopping point in your large project. At this point, you declare the task "complete" and move on to the next activity.

I can't tell you what a difference this strategy has made in my life and in the lives of many people who have attended my presentations. Try it! I'd love to receive an email from you to let me know how it works for you.

....

2. Learning to **move from your center of gravity (COG)** is not at all difficult. It does, however, involve learning to shift your weight from side to side while maintaining your erect posture (Alignment). Depending on how steady you are on your feet, you may require a bit of support or assistance. Practicing in a doorway gives you the option of support without you having to bend over to hold on to a countertop, which would throw off your balance and alignment.

HERE'S HOW!

- **Stand in the center of a door frame**. Have a chair behind you in case you need to sit down.

- Do the activity I taught you earlier in the section on Alignment: **Say or think the words, "Lengthen - Open - Make space in your chest."** Notice as your body gets taller and straighter, your neck and shoulder muscles relax, your shoulders drop down and back, and your chest expands. You can also say, "Tuck your Chin - let the crown of your head rise toward the ceiling."

- **Take a *conscious* breath** in through your nose, then exhale slowly with pursed lips, as I taught you in the section on Breathing.

- **Center yourself** by focusing on the activity you are about to begin. Try to avoid distractions.

- With your feet approximately hip-width apart, stay tall and *slowly* shift your weight to one side. (If you have one side that is stronger, shift to that side first.)

- Return to the middle (Center) starting position.

- *Slowly* shift your weight to the opposite side.

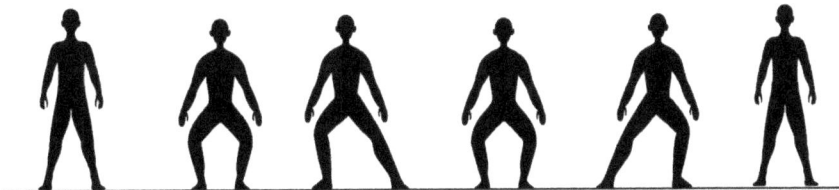

If it is safe, close your eyes during this exercise. It will improve your ability to sense where your body is in space (proprioception), which can enhance your capacity to balance. (We will do more activities in the chapter dedicated to balance a bit later in the book.)

....

3. **Holding objects close to your COG** is how you maintain leverage and keep from putting a strain on your back.

HERE'S HOW!

When you are lifting, moving, or toting something—such as carrying grocery bags, moving a piece of furniture, or even lifting and carrying a child or pet—always try to keep their weight as close to your COG as possible. (It's a little trickier carrying a child, because they will often be held on one side or another, but you can still think about keeping yourself well-aligned and the weight of the person close to your center of gravity.)

Getting familiar with your COG will allow you to learn to lift, move, walk, and carry with greater efficiency and ease. Together with good alignment, you can minimize putting undue stress on your hips, knees, or back, and possibly help your balance as well.

Overall, you want to strive to make The ABCs—Alignment, Breathing, and Centering—the foundation of everything you do. It takes some practice, I know. But once you get into the habit of doing them, you should notice the greater ease and confidence with which you move through the tasks of your daily life.

Using mindfulness and building on The ABCs, we will next explore the value and necessity of taking things a bit more slowly, to achieve the goal of aging safely, wisely, and well that we are seeking.

Chapter 3

Learning to Move in
S-L-O-W – M-O-T-I-O-N for
Mental and Physical Benefits

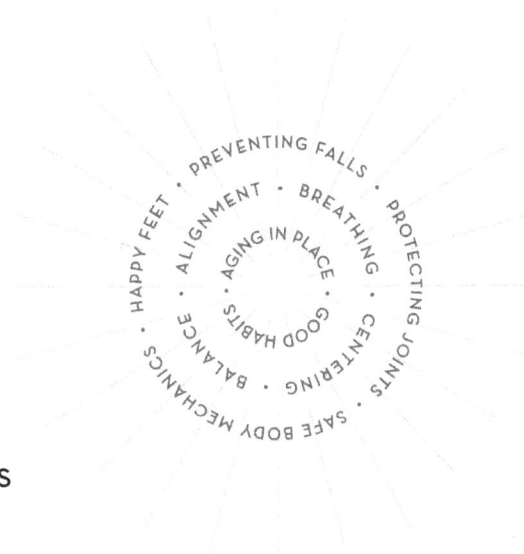

PREVENTING FALLS · PROTECTING JOINTS · SAFE BODY MECHANICS · BALANCE · CENTERING · GOOD HABITS · AGING IN PLACE · ALIGNMENT · BREATHING · HAPPY FEET

I n our fast-paced world, the prospect of moving in slow motion may sound next to impossible. Even if you're not immersed in a hurried environment, work schedule, or daily routine, you may simply have a tendency to do things too fast, run late, or hurry about as a habit. If you think these are habits you can't break, read on!

This chapter is all about slowing down—not in a way that makes you unproductive or ineffective, but actually the opposite. As you'll learn, the practice of simply taking your pace down a notch (or two, or three) can have significant mental and physical benefits.

Let's dip a foot in (slowly, of course), and find out how!

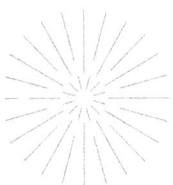

What Is It?

S-l-o-w–M-o-t-i-o-n is the third step in The ABC Mind-Body System. When you think of slow motion, your mind probably conjures an image of a movie, where the film speed intentionally causes a person or scene to move like molasses for a specific effect. This isn't quite what we're going for here, but we *are* talking about slowing your pace significantly so that you can feel and appreciate the difference between scurrying and walking with comfort, confidence, and a more balanced, even youthful, gait.

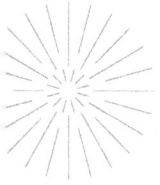

Why Is It Important?

As I said in the section on Mindfulness, slowing down offers both mental and physical benefits, as it allows you to become more conscious of your internal and external environments. Questions this might prompt are:

* Is my home or workplace set up so I can be safe and comfortable?

* Do I have pain or discomfort somewhere in my body?

* Am I tense and just need to breathe?

* Is there something I need to do to have greater peace of mind?

Becoming aware of these things can help you avoid potential accidents, injuries, and other challenges to your health and well-being. It can also help you determine if you need to have pain or discomfort checked out by a doctor or other healthcare professional, including a physical therapist.

Besides giving you time to reflect on your external and internal environments, slowing down also gives you time to think about actions you are considering taking. This is especially beneficial to those of us who tend to be somewhat impulsive. Have you ever made a bad decision or done something you regret because you acted in haste or on an impulse? I know I have in the past, but I eventually stopped letting anyone or anything rush me. It's not worth the risks!

Here's a tip that may help you slow down before taking an impulsive action or making an important decision:

* Count to 10 and do some conscious breathing before taking the action. That's one way to *slow down* and possibly avoid a costly mistake or accident before taking the action.

* Ask yourself: Is my solution to this challenge the best? Are there alternatives I might want to consider?

When you slow down and weigh your options, you may find you achieve more favorable outcomes than when you rush and make a hasty decision.

When doing physical activities, there are several benefits of using *S-l-o-w– M-o-t-i-o-n*:

* Slowing a movement down can help you develop strength, balance, and coordination, especially when you are just learning a new activity. Why? It gives the muscles time to develop the tone and control they require to do the activity.

* It gives you time to be mindful of what you're doing, and how you feel as you're doing it, so you can prevent a fall or injury.

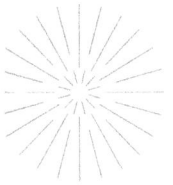

How Do You Achieve It?

Depending on how much of a speedster you tend to be—whether when walking, eating, talking, cleaning, or any other task at hand—simply think of slowing yourself down. I'll show you ways to do this in a moment, but first a reminder.

As with so many strategies in this book, you benefit more from each practice activity when you:

* Begin with an attitude of being willing to try. (We will explore the power of the words you speak to yourself in Chapter 5, but for now, just be willing to try.)

* Begin by *consciously* Aligning, Breathing, and Centering using the techniques you learned in Chapter 2: "**Lengthen – Open – Make space in your chest**" and "**Tuck your chin – Let the crown of your head rise toward the ceiling**"; slow, prolonged exhalations through pursed lips; and Start–Act–Stop.

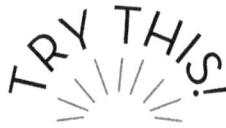

TRY THIS!

1. **Say the words "S-l-o-w-M-o-t-i-o-n" like one long word.** You may feel ridiculous doing it, but it works!

   I created this method while working with a patient learning to walk again. Despite his challenges, he insisted on walking fast, saying he couldn't slow down because he had always been a speedy walker, even though it jeopardized his safety and balance.

   Turning to face him, I said, "Okay, let's try this." In the most animated, exaggerated way I could manage, I opened my mouth wide and slowly enunciated the words, "S–L–O–W–M–O–T–I–O–N." Everyone around us laughed, including my patient.

   It took a minute before he gave in and tried the exercise. Then it took several tries before he was able to open his mouth wide and draw the words out. When he finally succeeded, we were both amazed. He actually walked more slowly with a better and safer gait!

Note that participants in my programs generally break up with laughter when we do this activity. Now it's your turn. If you want a good laugh, do this activity in front of a mirror. Laughing is good not only for your health but for your soul.

2. Practice Stand-to-Sit-to-Stand

This is one of the most important functional fitness activities you can do. Research has shown that your ability to sit and stand independently, without holding on to anything, is directly related to your ability to age safely and well.

- Begin this exercise by standing in front of a sturdy, straight-back chair. Make sure at least one of your legs is touching the edge of the seat behind you and your feet are approximately hip-width apart for good base of support (BOS).

- Moving as *slowly* as you can, press your hips back and down toward the seat of the chair. Your knees will begin to bend in preparation for sitting down (semi-squatting).

- Lower yourself only as far as you can before feeling you may lose control and "plop" down.

- Slowly return to erect standing by pressing your hips forward and straightening your knees.

- Strive to do this 3 to 10 times each time you need to get up or sit down throughout your day.

- Progress with this exercise until you can lower yourself to a fully seated position without plopping or needing to hold on to something for balance or support, and then be able to come to standing without needing support.

The ultimate goal here is being able to sit and stand from any seat without needing support. Just remember not to push your limits while doing this exercise—and don't hesitate to use arm-rests or a supportive device if you need it to be safe. **It's always safety first!**

What's great about this stand-to-sit exercise is that it can be done throughout the day, since sitting and standing are part of most people's everyday activities—and it's an excellent way to practice doing something in *S-l-o-w-M-o-t-i-o-n.*

Remember: Any activity you want to do to increase your strength, balance, and endurance should be done in "sets" of 3, 5, or 10 repetitions. (I recommend spacing these sets throughout your day so that you don't become sore or too fatigued to function the next day.) These are great numbers to commit to—so make sure you're getting those reps in.

Next, we will build on The ABCs in Chapter 2 by exploring another element of the 5-Step system: The Basic Moves. These will train you to use correct body mechanics so that you can bend, lift, carry things, and move more safely, wisely, and well—no matter your age!

Chapter 4

The Basic Moves
and the Principles of
Safe Body Mechanics

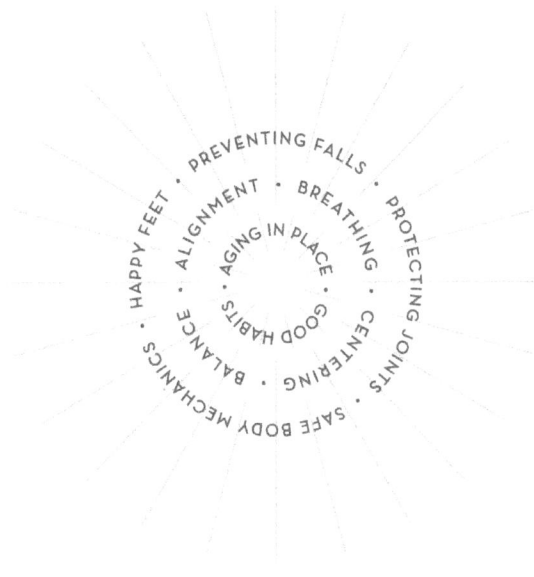

PREVENTING FALLS · PROTECTING JOINTS · CENTERING · SAFE BODY MECHANICS · BALANCE · GOOD HABITS · AGING IN PLACE · BREATHING · ALIGNMENT · HAPPY FEET

F or several years, I was the primary educator in back injury prevention at the prestigious Cedars-Sinai Medical Center in Los Angeles. In addition to teaching class participants The ABC System, I also instructed them in ten principles of safe bending, lifting, and carrying. One of those principles was to coordinate a heavy-lifting task with a second person.

As part of the training, I had two male staff members come to the front of the room to demonstrate by lifting a long, heavy table together. They were instructed to do The ABCs, look into each other's eyes, then do a slow count of three to synchronize their lift.

Well, either they weren't listening, or they decided they knew better. One of them mumbled a swift "1, 2, 3" then proceeded to lift the table without even looking at his partner. I cringed at the back injury waiting to happen!

I'm guessing that at least one time in your life, you've done something similarly reckless or unwitting—something that caused you to cry out in pain or say "My back just went out!" Whether the culprit was moving furniture, picking up a child, or simply grabbing a heavy grocery or tote bag at an awkward angle, it's a rare person who hasn't tweaked their back doing a simple, everyday task.

When I was new to being a physical therapist, I was shocked to see healthy, physically fit young men come to my department with back pain. I shouldn't have been surprised, though. I've encountered scores of healthy, fit men (and women) who think they can lift or move heavy objects with their brute strength alone. (Spoiler alert—you can't without risk of injury!)

In this chapter, I'm going to teach you the key skills for preventing unnecessary and unwanted pains, accidents, and injuries—to yourself *and* possibly to others—by getting you savvy with the basic moves and principles of safe bending, lifting, and carrying.

What Are They?

The Basic Moves are a series of movements that involve squatting, lifting, and stepping activities. They train you to use correct body mechanics, which encompass how you bend, lift, and carry objects—or transfer patients, if you are a caregiver or work in a healthcare setting. They provide the safest, most efficient way to perform any back-threatening tasks.

Why Are They Important?

Simply put, The Basic Moves strengthen your ability to keep correct alignment as you go about your daily activities. Statistics show that most back pain can be traced to the use of poor body mechanics. Healthcare workers are particularly affected by back pain and injuries, so if you work in this field, these techniques will be especially helpful for you, but they definitely apply to everyone. Your safety, and the safety of the person you may be helping, are at risk if you do not use the correct body mechanics taught in this chapter. So please take them seriously so you can prevent unnecessary pain, injury, or even harm.

The Basic Moves also encourage the use and strengthening of the muscles designed for bending and lifting: the buttocks (gluteus maximus), which is responsible for controlling your hips as you bend and lift from a squat position; thigh muscles (quadriceps), which control your knees' ability to bend and straighten; and the core muscles we discussed in the section on Alignment (and will discuss further in Chapter 6), which are the deep muscles that surround your torso. If you need a visual, the following video demonstrates the anatomical details for how to properly do a squat:

https://www.muscleandmotion.com/full-squat-anatomy/

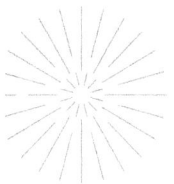

How Do You Achieve Them?

Here comes the fun part! There are four Basic Moves, and I can't emphasize enough how much you will benefit from learning to do them correctly. Before we get to them, though, let's go over a few important tips:

* It can be helpful to **get these movements right** by looking at yourself in a full-length mirror, or having someone watch you as you practice. If certain conditions, such as joint limitations, make the moves a little more challenging, simply do the best you can.

* For some women in my programs, they resist **doing squats correctly** because it doesn't look particularly "feminine." But to do them right,

you need to stick your butt out and take a wide stance, like a football player in a huddle—so forget about looking "ladylike" for this one.

* Remember that every activity we do in this book begins with **Aligning** ("Lengthen – Open – Make space in your chest" and "Tuck your chin – Let the crown of your head rise toward the ceiling"), *Conscious* **Breathing**, and **Centering** (focusing on one activity at a time so that your mind and body are working together).

* After doing your ABCs, remember that each move begins by **moving from your physical Center** (COG), which is just below your belly button when you are standing.

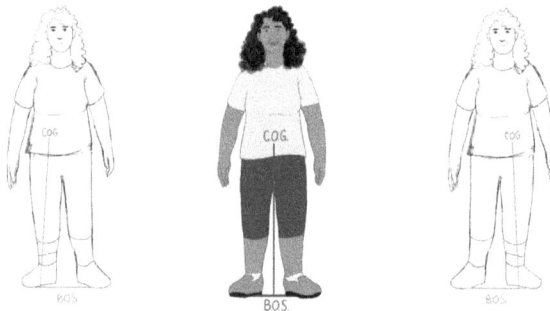

- All The Basic Moves **require some degree of balance**. A simple definition of *balance* is the ability to keep an object's, or a person's, center of gravity (COG) over their base of support (BOS). In humans, that BOS is the area between our two feet, no matter how close or far apart they may be. **During The Basic Moves, your COG is always positioned over your BOS for better balance and control.** (As a reminder, understanding and managing your balance will be covered in Chapter 7, related to preventing falls and injuries.)

- The **weight-shifting, stepping, and walking movements** in The Basic Moves are about learning how to shift and move your weight (COG) as you are carrying something, or someone, in what therapists call a "transfer." Said another way, it is about the transition of your pelvis over each leg as you lift, move, or carry in any direction.

This brief video is advanced for most readers, but it is an excellent one to show good body mechanics when preparing for the moves that follow, and for squats in general:

https://bit.ly/good-body-mechanics

1. Squat-Stand

Front View   *Side View*

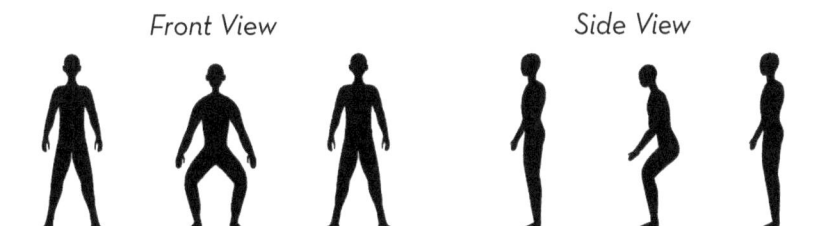

1. Begin with your ABCs in an erect standing position, with feet at least hip-width apart for good BOS.

2. Press your hips back, and let your knees bend, keeping them behind your toes.

3. Keep your head, neck, and trunk aligned as you lower down into the squat. (Imagine the position of football players when they are squatted in a huddle.)

4. Return to standing by pressing your hips forward and your knees back. to your starting position.

2. Squat-Shift

Front / Back View

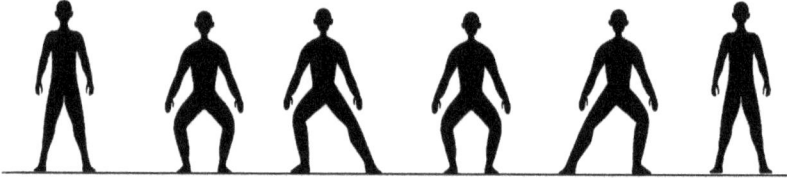

1. Return to the squat position.

2. In *S-l-o-w-M-o-t-i-o-n*, keeping your trunk lengthened, and maintaining *conscious* breathing, move your COG over one leg so that the opposite leg is straightened and your weight is mostly on the opposite foot. Note: If there is a difference in strength between your right and left sides, go to your stronger side first.

3. Slowly glide your hips back to the Centered squat position.

4. Without straightening up to a standing position, glide your hips to the other side. You will feel this in your buttock and thigh muscles if you are doing it right.

5. Return to Center and then to standing.

6. Note: Use the back of a chair for balance if you need it. Again, safety first!

3. Squat-Shift-Step

Front / Back View

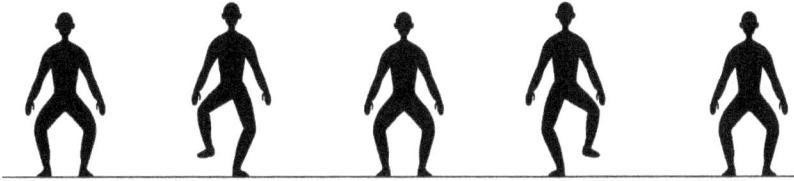

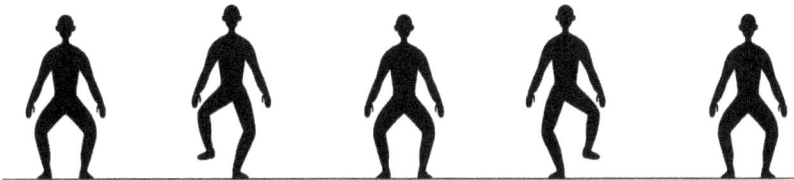

1. Return to the squat position and remain there as you do the following moves. (Don't forget to maintain a lengthened spine for Alignment.)

2. If you can do it safely, take several steps to one side, and stay squatted as you return to center. Then do the same stepping to the other side. Remember to go to your strong side first. Repeat this several times before standing straight again.

4. Squat-Shift-Walk Around

Front / Back View

This Basic Move gets a lot of laughs, but it's the most important.

1. Return to the squat position.

2. This time, you're going to walk in different directions, including circles. (It helps to imagine a Sumo wrestler stance as he is stepping around the mat—forward, backward, sideways, diagonally, etc.)

3. Return to erect standing position when you or your muscles fatigue. *You always want to listen to your body.*

Now, you may be asking, "Why should I do these silly-looking activities?"

That is a great question—and I have a great answer!

Your ability to safely lift, carry, move, and transfer people or objects is directly related to your ability to do the above basic movements correctly.

QUESTIONS AND TIPS FOR PROPER SQUATTING, LIFTING, AND MOVING

1. Assess the lifting or moving task you are about to do, then ask yourself:

    *   Is it safe for me to do? Should I ask someone else to do it instead?

    *   Does it require two or more people to accomplish?

2. If you're doing the task alone:

    A. Prepare with your ABCs: Align – Breathe – Center.

    B. Stand with a wide base of support, and be prepared to step in the direction of the move.

    C. Squat correctly, by bending at the hips and knees, while keeping your spine well-aligned. Keep your knees behind your toes unless doing a deep squat.

    D. Hold whatever you are lifting or moving as close to your COG as possible.

E. Push, don't pull. This allows you to use your body weight to move the item/person and reduces the risk of falling.

F. Divide the load into two parts to avoid lifting something that causes you to lean backward.

G. Avoid a combination of bending, lifting, and twisting moves. Use the Basic Moves technique #4—Squat-Shift-Walk Around—in the direction you want to move, or to transfer something or someone.

3. If you're doing the task with others:

A. Plan ahead, as above.

B. Prepare with your ABCs: Align – Breathe – Center.

C. Observe each other for correct positioning before doing the lift or transfer.

D. Do a slow count to 3 in preparation for the lift or transfer. (Remember the story I told you at the beginning of the chapter about the two men lifting a heavy table, where one didn't wait to synchronize with the other? Be sure not to do that!)

E. Perform the lift or transfer *slowly* and *with control.* This way, you can stop if necessary.

F. Clearly communicate with everyone involved in the lift or transfer.

G. Avoid the combination of bending, lifting, and twisting. Again, use The Basic Moves technique #4—Squat-Shift-Walk Around—in the direction you want to move.

H. Healthcare workers and professionals may use equipment to help move objects or people, but the principles of using good body mechanics still apply.

Now that you have learned the principles of safe body mechanics and The Basic Moves, you might enjoy the 16-minute video I did in 2000 that lays out the original ABC system. The participants in the class were friends and associates, and you'll get to see a younger me as well as the old CRT monitors we used.

https://bit.ly/ABCs-2000-video

In the next chapter, we're going to explore another set of ABC(S): four qualities that will be pivotal in your journey of personal growth and transformation.

Chapter 5

The ABC(S) of Personal Growth and Transformation: Attitudes, Beliefs, Commitment, and Self-Talk

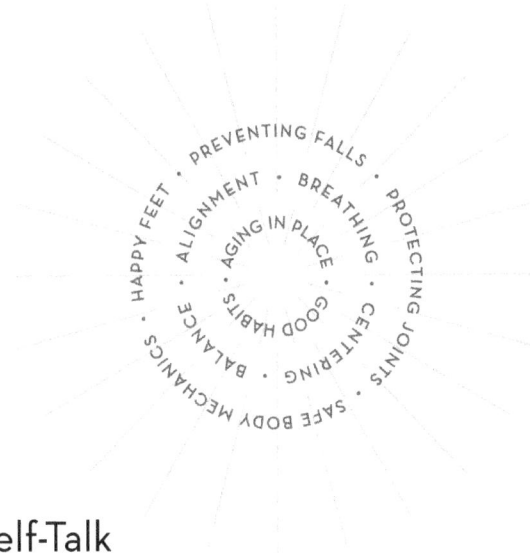

The circular text reads: PREVENTING FALLS · PROTECTING JOINTS · CENTERING · GOOD HABITS · AGING IN PLACE · BREATHING · ALIGNMENT · HAPPY FEET · SAFE BODY MECHANICS · BALANCE

My first version of The ABC System focused primarily on physical movement and performance. The idea was, and still is, that by learning to Align, Breathe, and Center, you can improve how you look, feel, and function. After some time, I realized that a second set of ABCs was necessary for managing our mental well-being: Attitudes, Beliefs, and Commitment—with the additional "S" referring to Self-Talk. (You got a taste of self-talk when you learned to "Lengthen, Open," etc., but we will go more in depth here.)

While all the chapters of this book have immense value, this chapter may be the most powerful, because none of what I've taught you thus far will have significant impact for you if your mindset is one of "I can't," "I shouldn't," or "What will they think?" or if you don't make a commitment to do the work that will allow for the transformation you are striving for.

What follows are my definitions, descriptions, and examples of these ABC(S), which I hope will give you some direction in sorting out your own mindset elements, determining which are useful for you to hold on to, and which might best be set free. Ultimately, the goal is for you to be, do, and have the things that give your life the most joy, purpose, and meaning.

As you will see, there is an intimate relationship between beliefs and attitudes. Learning to distinguish the difference between them, and how and why to consider changing any of them, can be a potentially rewarding challenge.

ATTITUDES

By definition, *attitude* is a mental position, feeling, or emotion toward a fact or condition. However, I see the definition of "attitude" as more of a *reaction* to something you believe is right or wrong, good or bad. (I told you beliefs and attitudes were interrelated!) Whether the reaction is immediate or takes time to develop and brew inside you, it is a reflection of how you interpreted something that happened or was said. In short, you gave that something a specific meaning, and now you have a reaction to it.

I recently experienced an example of this when someone made a mistake on my lunch order. While I'm exaggerating to make a point, I found myself in my *belief* that it's wrong to make a mistake on someone's food order. My *reaction* to that belief became a choice I had to make: become self-righteous and display a nasty, negative attitude as I confronted the server, or choose to be friendly as I brought the mistake to her attention and asked for my order to be fixed.

What doesn't change in this scenario is my order being wrong. What *can* change is my attitude and how I go about remedying the situation. Either way, my attitude—whether positive or negative—will get my lunch order corrected, but the more positive one will create less stress within me as well as for the server, leaving us both happier.

Another way to look at it is that attitude is a mental outlook or emotion about a circumstance or condition in your life, your community, or even the world. Typically, it is either positive or negative, constructive or destructive, and it is changeable if you *decide* to interpret a situation differently. Optimism and pessimism are examples of general attitudes that impact how you view life and its possibilities. Which one do you think yields better results in your life?

The good news is that with mindfulness, intention, and just a little effort, you can *choose to change* that negative attitude, especially if it is not producing the results you want. You may even know someone who has the ability to view almost everything with a positive attitude; despite challenges, they choose to see a "Higher Power," if you believe in one, "working in their favor." For those who have a less-than-positive attitude, this optimistic outlook may be an annoyance (after all, misery loves company). But you don't have to look far to see that those who exude a positive attitude are generally happier and have better relationships and quality of life than those who don't. Being with an optimistic person also tends to improve our own sense of mental and physical well-being.

Check out these examples of negative and positive attitudes.

Negative Attitude

"I can't do this. It's too much work and it probably won't make a difference."

"Some of these moves will be too difficult for me. Why bother even trying them?"

"It seems like a lot. I don't want to put in that much effort."

"I don't want to change my routine, and I have too many problems to fix anyway."

Can you feel the defeastist vibe?

Now let's look at a person who has a more constructive perspective.

Positive Attitude

"I've never done any of these moves before, but I'm willing to give them a try."

"I can't wait to see how I can improve my mobility and balance by practicing these activities."

"I knew some of the things in this book, but I learned a lot too, and now I really feel like I can stay fit and independent for the rest of my life."

"I'm excited to make time for these exercises and to notice my triggers. It's going to be fun!"

What a difference, right? Do you see how these positive statements are really more about perspective? You can believe something ("these won't work for me," "I'm too old to change at this point"), but in an instant, you can decide/choose to have the opposite outlook, regardless of what you may believe. And I can tell you from experience, that shift to a more optimistic/positive perspective goes a long way in promoting better health and fitness—and can even change someone's belief entirely.

As a last note, one of the best attitudes of all is one of gratitude. Focusing on the things in your life for which you are grateful can be transformative for your mind and body. So, choose to be empowered by an attitude that favors optimism and positivity!

BELIEFS

A belief is simply something you embrace as fact. Let me say that again. *A belief is something you embrace as fact.* This doesn't mean the belief is necessarily something true; it merely means you *believe* it to be true.

Whether your beliefs are the result of the culture(s) into which you were born or raised, your family's religion, ethnic, or national identity, messaging from the media, past experiences, the list goes on, they can have serious implications for what you think is possible for yourself, others, and even the world. In the same way your attitude influences what you think is or isn't possible, beliefs can also produce positive or negative results in your life. And yes, choosing to change an ingrained belief can be challenging, but the results are often worth the effort.

So, as we did with attitude, I'm going to present you with two sets of belief statements. But this time, we're going to contrast the less empowering one with one that frees you to realize your dreams and potential.

Less Empowering Belief

"Women aren't as smart in certain subjects as men."

"Strong men shouldn't show emotion."

"I'm too old to be considered beautiful/handsome."

"It's too late for me to get into better shape."

These, among too many others, tend to cut deeply into our sense of ourselves and limit what we see possible in our lives.

Now let's look at a person who is willing to change those ingrained beliefs.

Positive New Belief

"Women excel in all arenas that men do."

"Strong men are confident in showing their feelings."

"I am uniquely beautiful/handsome at every age."

"It's never too late for me to get into better shape."

Consider if you have any beliefs like these. It's worth taking the time to explore them and decide if it's worth making some changes.

Simply believing that you can change something you've always believed to be true, or that past experiences have dictated, changes your biochemistry—especially when you say it out loud. Speak these four statements and you'll see what I mean. And yes, I do realize there are many more ingrained beliefs than these that could be holding you back. The point is that with awareness and intention to achieve your life goals, beliefs can be changed. In the case of striving to improve your level of fitness and well-being, you make the new belief a reality by proving it to yourself through your actions.

COMMITMENT

Now that we've explored Attitudes and Beliefs—and you've hopefully gotten some ideas for a few you'd like to shift—we arrive at the subject of Commitment. After all, what is the point of deciding to make changes if you're not willing to commit to them?

Look, I get it. It's easy to read a book or join a program and see all the possibilities in it. It's also common for that initial excitement to wane, or for the early dedication to get overshadowed by, well, life. We start out gung ho, maybe even with concrete goals, and then we lapse back into our old routine, or get busy with work, or don't see results fast enough so we give up.

I don't have to tell you that if you give up on a commitment, you won't see results. There are certainly times to let a commitment go—like when you overcommit and learn to start saying no when you're asked for the twentieth time to volunteer for some event! But in general, if you want to see real change in your life, no matter the area, it requires commitment on your part to see it through.

Nothing is a magic bullet; good Alignment, *conscious* Breathing, Centering, learning to use *S-l-o-w–M-o-t-i-o-n*, and mastering The Basic Moves . . . none of those things will improve if you don't commit to learning the techniques and practicing them consistently. In short, without Commitment, your knowledge—and even your transformed Attitudes and Beliefs—won't amount to a hill of beans.

Ideally, you will be eager to learn the activities I've taught you and to incorporate them into your daily and/or weekly life until they become part of your routine.

For example:

* If you catch yourself sitting or standing with slouched posture, you remember The ABCs, realign yourself immediately, and go about your business. My experience is that after a while, the better posture becomes a new habit as your body starts looking, feeling, and even functioning better.

* As you start becoming conscious of your breathing, periodically stop and take a deep diaphragmatic breath with a slow, prolonged exhalation, then go about your business. Once more, you turn to this technique because you find it de-stresses you and gives you more energy. In other words, it has become a new habit!

* Need to pick someone or something up? When you start to bend in your usual way, you remember to use *S-l-o-w–M-o-t-i-o-n* and The

Basic Moves so that you avoid back pain. After a while, it too becomes a habit as you transform the ways you move through life by weaving The ABC Mind-Body System into it.

If you prefer a more organized and structured approach to making commitments, my friend Stacey has found the following advice can be incredibly helpful, especially if you feel overwhelmed with all the recommended activities and the possible introduction of new habits.

With this approach, you don't make a long-term commitment to any of the practices in this book. If you think you have to do something for weeks, months, or years, you likely won't do it. Instead, commit to **one week**. That's it. During this period, you get acquainted with and use an activity you choose— and hopefully see and feel the positive results of doing it.

If this technique appeals to you, here are some suggestions:

* Focus on being mindful for one week.

* Visualize, for at least two minutes a day, one aspect of your life you'd like to improve. Picture yourself walking more steadily, breathing more deeply, sitting and standing with ease . . . anything you'd like to be able to do with more confidence and strength than you are now.

* Observe your posture while sitting, standing and walking. That's it. Just your posture.

* When you have to lift, move, or carry something, remember to use S-l-o-w—M-o-t-i-o-n and The Basic Moves.

* Practice *conscious* breathing sessions three to four times a day, for as many repetitions as you can (using the guidance in Chapter 2).

* Use the Start–Act–Stop technique whenever you do a task at home or at work.

* Monitor your attitude for one week. Nothing but your attitude. Notice if you tend to lean negative or positive. If you lean negative, see if you can flip your perspective to one that's more positive. Notice the difference it makes within and around you.

* Assess your beliefs about who you are, and what you can, cannot, should, and should not do. For those negative beliefs, write a new one that cancels it with "I can" or "I believe" statements. Notice how that changes your sense of yourself and what's possible in your life.

Can you see how manageable it feels to choose only *one* new practice or activity to try? And everyone can commit to doing something for one week. One new practice / attitude / belief for a week. That's it!

The beauty of this system is that it is *your* choice to re-up your commitment or not—or even to add a second (or third) practice or not—as the weeks go on. With this method, you're committing to making a change **but on your terms**. Each one-week mark gives you the chance to evaluate and decide. You are empowered not merely because you *think* you should do these things for your health and well-being, but because you actually *see* and *feel* the results. Before you know it, the new activity has become part of your everyday routine because it's making a positive difference in how you move, feel, and approach your life.

SELF-TALK

It's part of being human to talk to ourselves, whether in our heads or out loud—but it's the *type* of words and phrases we use during our self-talk that matters. For example, self-talk can be helpful for remembering things or getting organized, but not so helpful when it consists of phrases that are negative, limiting, and disempowering.

As we've discussed with Attitudes and Beliefs, words carry power over both our minds and bodies. So it's no surprise that when you say things like, "I *can't* [fill in the blank]," or "*I'll never be* as good as so and so at that," or "I *should* be more like so and so" or "I'm *not* worthy"... the list goes on and on... something unwanted happens. You may experience a loss of confidence in your ability to make good decisions, to take appropriate actions, or to simply be the person you want to be, all because you allow yourself to be limited in who you are and what you can do or be.

The good news is that you can shift this habit by becoming mindful of your negative "self-talk." Here are simple ways you can do it:

* Decide here and now that you will never again speak negative words to yourself, or use negative words to describe yourself to others. If you start to do it, catch yourself immediately and stop. In that moment, substitute an empowering expression, sometimes referred to as a "suggestion," like:

  • "I am healthy, strong, and wise."
  • "I am an expression of love and tolerance."
  • "I am confident and open to learning new things."

* Take a few moments to identify and even write down the negative things you think or say about yourself, such as "Nobody loves me" or "I'm such a failure." Next, find a way to say the opposite, such as "I am lovable and enjoy sharing my love with others" or "I'm capable of anything I put my mind to."

* Another approach is to ask yourself, "Would I say these demeaning words to someone I love and respect, or to my child, grandchild, or best friend?" If the answer is no, then they are off the table for you too!

While I am not a trained psychologist, I've had enough life experience and have worked with enough mental health professionals to know that employing positive self-talk can completely change a person's life. I've seen it countless times in my work, and some of the results have been truly miraculous.

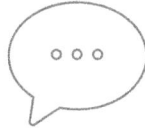

○ ○ ○

While I was working at Cedars-Sinai, an elderly lady was wheeled into the physical therapy gym with her two adult daughters at her side. She was there to make her first attempt at standing after having had surgery for her broken hip.

The poor woman was petrified with fear about trying to stand up between the parallel bars. She kept crying, "I can't, I can't, I can't!" That phrase had become her mantra.

Now, I was an excellent physical therapist with a multitude of strategies to help people overcome physical, and even mental, resistance to doing their exercises. But on that day, none of my strategies was good enough to take this woman past "I can't." Even with her daughters' prodding and encouragement, there was no getting her over her negative self-talk. For one of the only times in my professional career, I gave up.

"Okay," I said to her, "you win. I'm not going to try to make you stand."

This wasn't another strategy. I was serious—with one condition.

"I'm going to let you return to your room," I said, "but I want you to say the words 'I'll try' before I let you go."

After several more "I can'ts," I suddenly heard, in a barely audible voice, "I'll try."

As promised, rather than trying to make her stand again, I began to unlock her wheelchair brakes to send her back to her room. Then I stopped. Without any expectation, I leaned down and looked at her with a smile. "Would you like to try to stand?"

This next part of the story always gives me chills. Without a word, she let me put my arms around her for support. The woman not only stood, but she began *walking*. She walked the full length of the parallel bars, turned, and walked back again before sitting down.

That's the power of our "self-talk!"

....

That day taught me a lesson I will never forget. I already believed in the power of words to disempower or encourage, but after that, I began calling "should" and "can't" *forbidden words*. ("Don't 'should' on me and I won't 'should' on you" are favorite lyrics from a David Roth song. You'll find it on his album, *Rising in Love*.)

And while we're on the topic of "should," negative stereotypes are another potentially limiting factor about what we imagine is possible in our lives, or in the lives of others, based on what someone "should" or "should not" do at a certain age, or in certain circumstances. Can we agree to eliminate those right now too?

Listen, I understand that you may have grown up being criticized, or talked down to, or teased, and I know those tracks get laid pretty deep. But that doesn't mean those tracks can't be rewired. I can't tell you how many patients I've had who had difficulty walking and were handicapped by a fear of falling, yet were able to overcome that fear by simply saying words like, "I am tall, strong, and confident."

Are you beginning to sense the transformation this mind-body technique can make in your life and relationships? Consider teaching it to others in your life so they can benefit from your wisdom too.

TRY THIS!

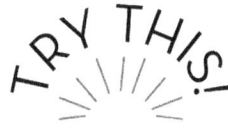

Add some of the following words and phrases into your daily self-talk vocabulary and see if you don't feel more empowered and experience positive differences:

- I am strong.

- I have perfect health.

- I have a sharp mind.

- I appreciate my body.

- I am confident and capable.

- I have excellent mobility.

- I can overcome any obstacle placed before me.

- I am beautiful/handsome as I am.

- I can change anything in my life I put my mind to.

- I learn new things with ease.

- I have gifts unique only to me (and I love them!)

- I appreciate my abilities and talents.

- I love myself.

Now it's your turn to add to this list. Take some time to identify what empowers you. What words have made a difference in the way you feel, see the world, and meet challenges? You may be pleasantly surprised at what a difference your self-talk can make in your life, and the lives of those around you.

Chapter 6

The Elements of Basic Physical Fitness: Building Blocks for Your Transformation

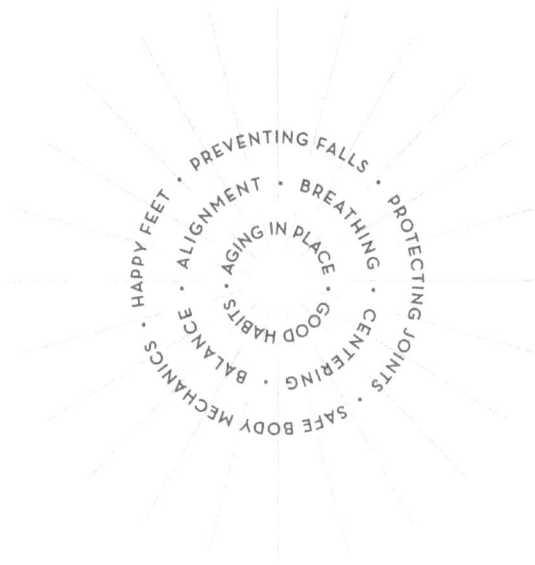

N ow that you're empowered with techniques for successful transformation, both sets of ABCs, the benefits of *S-l-o-w–M-o-t-i-o-n*, and The Basic Moves and principles of safe body mechanics, let's discuss the elements of basic physical fitness: flexibility, strength, endurance, core conditioning, and functional fitness. Having knowledge of these five components is a vital part of your fitness routine and will serve as additional building blocks for your transformation.

FLEXIBILITY

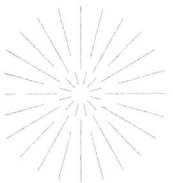

What Is It?

Flexibility refers to the capacity of each of the six types of movable joints in your body to go through their full ranges of motion.

Why Is It Important?

Flexibility, and full ranges of motion, are what enable you to:

* reach your arms up from your shoulder joint

* do squats, which require flexibility in your hip and knee joints

* turn your head, which occurs between your skull and cervical vertebrae

* bend to put on socks and shoes, which requires a mobile spine

* and more!

Even the ability of your chest to expand as you inhale and retract as you exhale requires flexibility of the ribs as they expand and contract from their attachments at the spine.

For a visual, imagine a door that has well-aligned hinges. It opens all the way and closes without squeaking and will probably last a long time. But if the hinges are out of alignment, the door will be unable to open and close all the way, will probably squeak, and will almost certainly break down eventually. While the movements of the joints in your body are generally more complex than the simple hinges of a door—besides bending and extending, they also perform some degree of sliding, gliding, or rotation, as you will see a little further on—you get the idea.

Think about your own body. Is there a particular joint (or joints) causing you pain and limited function? Perhaps you have arthritis, stiffness, or poor postural habits that have caused you to have restricted joint motion. These are the places you want to focus on most, with the aim of alleviating or restoring your limited range of motion.

The Alignment portion of The ABC Mind-Body System aims to ensure that all your joints are well-positioned for optimum safety, comfort, and performance. Strength is also a factor in you achieving these tasks, which we will discuss in the next section.

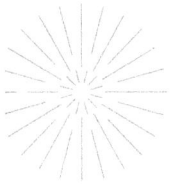

How Do You Achieve It?

The technique for increasing a joint's range of motion, no matter what caused its limitation, is **stretching**.

An important consideration when you want to increase the range of motion of your shoulder joint is to know the difference between the shoulder *girdle* and shoulder *joint*.

The **shoulder girdle** enables the movements of shrugging your shoulders towards your ears (elevation), and pressing them down again (depression), as well as rolling your shoulders forward (protraction) and rolling them back (retraction).

The **shoulder joint** allows you to raise your arm(s) over your head (flexion), down and back (extension), out to the side, away from your body (abduction), and down or back toward your body (adduction).

While it is true that the shoulder girdle has to move to help the shoulder joint get to its full range of motion, too often people substitute shoulder girdle motion for shoulder joint motion.

Caution: No matter what type of stretching you're doing, avoid doing stretching exercises in joints that are too flexible (hypermobile). That can lead to pain, loss of stability of the joints, and actual loss of function.

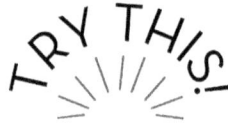

TRY THIS!

1. Sit or stand in front of a mirror.

2. Raise your arm 90 degrees straight out in front of you or straight out to the side. If you have limited strength or range in your shoulder joint, your shoulder girdle will rise up as you try to lift your arm. Note that you can lift only about 45 degrees strictly from your shoulder joint.

3. The shoulder joint and shoulder girdle work in synergy when you reach up to higher levels. Can you see that when you try to lift your arm(s) higher?

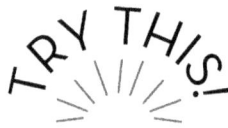

TRY THIS!

The following stretching technique is based on yoga. It provides the safest way to stretch, particularly because breathing is integral to it.

1. Begin with the foundational ABCs by getting into **Alignment** (your best lengthened posture), doing *conscious* **Breathing**, and **Centering** yourself by being focused on the activity.

2. Move the body part to be stretched into its "lengthened" position. For example, if you are stretching your shoulder joint, hold out your arm the best you can, either to the front or out to the side, and control your shoulder girdle.

3. Hold that position for a s-l-o-w count of three, maintaining a steady breathing pattern.

4. Take a deep diaphragmatic breath in through your nose and slowly move into a more stretched or lengthened position as you exhale.

5. **Avoid bouncing.**

6. Repeat 3 to 5 times. You will probably have achieved your maximum stretch by the last repetition.

Important note: Stretching comes with some discomfort as you reach and move farther into the stretched position. However, there is a difference between "discomfort" and "pain." Moves that are good for you often feel better when they are repeated. If the pain or discomfort gets worse as you repeat a move, *listen to your body and stop right away.*

Last, you may have heard the terms "static" and "dynamic" stretching. The technique described above is considered "static" because you are *holding* a position. "Dynamic" stretching has you moving in and out of a position, like swinging your arms up and down, or kicking your leg up and down. While dynamic stretching may require greater balance and general conditioning, it's good for you to be aware of the two approaches to increasing your flexibility.

STRENGTH

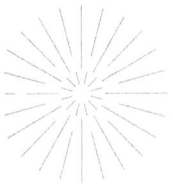

What Is It?

Strength is the ability of your voluntary muscles—those that move your face, head, neck, trunk, arms, and legs—to contract to move your joints and to exert the force needed to perform activities.

(Note here that *strength* and *power* are not synonymous. Power requires overcoming a weight, or some form of resistance, with speed and multiple repetitions. It's true that each of your everyday activities requires a certain amount of speed to coordinate the activity; however, speed has no bearing on strength. You could bend your elbow one hundred times, at any speed, but you only increase power if you add weights (resistance) and enough repetitions to fatigue the muscles you are using.)

To be clear, if you are able to lift your body and its parts, you have *strength*, regardless of how much effort it takes to do the movement.

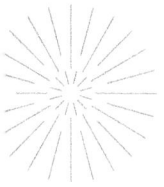

Why Is It Important?

You want to have enough strength to perform your everyday activities—from getting in and out of bed, to enjoying your favorite hobby or sport, to doing heavy construction work, and everything in between—without struggling or becoming fatigued before you complete a task.

If you are a healthcare worker or caregiver who must do a lot of lifting, that task requires not only strength but good body mechanics as well (those you learned in The Basic Moves chapter).

Research shows that there are also mental and physical benefits to developing your strength beyond what you need for your everyday activities. Those benefits include:

* Improved weight-management metabolism, as toned muscles use more calories

* Improved bone, joint, and muscle health, which is especially useful for many arthritic and osteoporotic conditions

* Improved mood and relief of depression

* Possibly even increased longevity

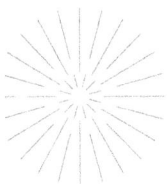

How Do You Achieve It?

The general principle for strengthening muscles is to make them work against resistance or overcome a force. Your own body weight provides natural resistance, as it works to overcome the force of gravity. (Think of how your leg, back, and arm muscles work when you bend over and pick something or someone up.)

You can increase your strength by adding weights or resistance bands to everyday activities. For example, when you are sitting or standing, you can hold a weight or resistance band as you practice raising your arm(s) over your head, out to the side, or in a diagonal/rotational move across your body. You can purchase comfortable weights to hold in your hand that begin at one pound, then two, three, five, and ten. Even using light weights that are manageable for you, then working toward the next level (such as moving from 2-lb weights to 3-lb weights), will increase your strength and endurance, as will adding repetitions (the number of times you repeat a movement).

Do be aware that this book is not about providing you with a specific "exercise" routine, but rather an understanding of safe and effective movement. With that in mind, on the next page is a brief list of ideas you may want to use to create a routine that suits your abilities and goals. There are also plentiful demonstrations online and in books to teach you moves that are safe and beneficial for your physical fitness and function. Just remember to integrate your ABCs into them! And always listen to your body for any signs or symptoms that a particular activity is not the safest or most beneficial for you.

*   bicep curls (either sitting or standing) – for lifting and carrying things
*   shoulder and/or tricep presses – for pushing up from a chair or using a cane or walker
*   arm lifts – for putting something on an upper shelf or combing your hair

DID YOU KNOW?

Muscles work in three different ways, depending on the activity you are doing. For example, the bicep muscle in your upper arm shortens (concentric contraction) as it does an activity like picking up a book. As you lower the book, it lengthens (eccentric contraction) to keep your arm from dropping down. When you hold the book still, in any position, it is called an "isometric" contraction.

THE VALUE OF ISOMETRICS

An isometric activity is one where muscles tense, or tighten, without getting longer or shorter. They can be highly effective as a strengthening technique. What's great is that you can perform isometric activities anywhere, with no weights needed.

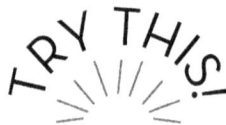

TRY THIS!

1. Choose a single muscle, like the bicep in your upper arm, or a group of muscles, like those when you do the Foot Press exercise (pg. 85).

2. Do your steady, *conscious* Breathing as you progressively tense and then hold the tension in these muscles. **This is especially important** because you may have a tendency to hold your breath while doing an isometric, or any activity that requires you to strain or exert a lot of force. Holding your breath while straining is potentially dangerous because it tends to increase blood pressure, which could lead to a heart attack or stroke. So, whether you're doing isometrics or straining while doing a task, START CONSCIOUS BREATHING AT THE OUTSET.

   As a helpful aid, anytime you are going to be exerting a lot of force, or "straining" during an activity, begin the activity by **counting**, **humming**, **singing**, or **talking out loud**, anything that ensures you are not holding your breath.

3. Now, build the isometric for as long as you can, while maintaining a steady Breathing pattern.

4. When you can hold the tension no longer, release the muscle(s) slowly and shake them out to relax them.

5. As with every technique you are learning here, strive to integrate it into your everyday activities.

ENDURANCE

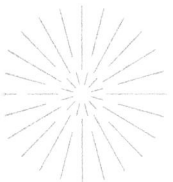

What Is It?

Endurance encompasses your ability to do an activity for a sustained time before fatiguing. It relates to your aerobic capacity, which is measured by your heart's ability to maintain a predetermined heart rate for a certain amount of time. There are tables that offer guidelines, but any aerobic or cardiac conditioning should be planned with your healthcare provider or fitness consultant.

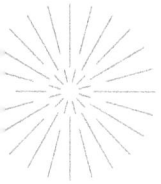

Why Is It Important?

If you lack endurance, you may find yourself running out of steam as you move through your day, or not have enough energy to walk to your mailbox and back, or through the aisles of your favorite store, or even find it challenging to raise your arm the number of times needed to comb your hair. (Okay, maybe that last one is a poor example, since some of us older adults don't have that much hair anymore!) But seriously, none of us wants to lose energy while doing even the most menial of tasks, let alone those that require more exertion. This is why you want to do what you can to maintain optimal endurance.

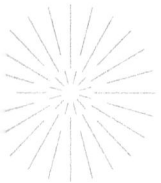

How Do You Achieve It?

Your endurance depends largely on having a healthy heart, lungs, and neuromuscular system. So unless you have a medically limiting condition that is worsened by increasing your activity level, you are encouraged to build or increase your endurance.

How do you do it? Simply extend the length of time you perform any physical activity, or the number of times (repetitions) you do it. And it doesn't have to be complicated. Walk a little farther; sit and stand several times before you walk away from a chair; lift a can of beans or tomatoes several times before you open it. All of those little additions to everyday tasks build endurance. And if you have the capacity to take it a bit further, do it.

You can:

* Practice the basic moves 10 times in a row instead of 5, then repeat 2 to 3 times as you're able.

* Walk to the mailbox then back, then back out to the mailbox to retrieve the mail, so that you make two round trips instead of one.

* Walk to the end of your driveway and back . . . then repeat, aiming to work up to 5 trips.

* Swim one lap. Work your way to two, then more if you can.

You get the picture. Do note that it's often a good idea to be medically evaluated by your personal physician, then develop a specific fitness program in coordination with a physical therapist or fitness professional.

This is also a perfect time to set what are called SMART goals—Specific, Measurable, Achievable, Relevant, and Time-bound. They can help you achieve the transformation we keep talking about.

If you're unfamiliar with SMART goals, here's a brief breakdown of the key elements:

Specific: goals are clear and well-defined, leaving no room for misinterpretation by identifying exactly what needs to be accomplished.

Measurable: goals are quantifiable, allowing progress to be tracked and measured, which helps you stay focused and motivated.

Achievable: goals are realistic and attainable, taking into account the resources and constraints available.

Relevant: goals align with your values, needs, and priorities.

Time-Bound: goals have a specific deadline or time frame for completion, providing a sense of urgency and focus.

The benefits of SMART goals are:

* Increased clarity and focus

* Improved motivation and accountability

* Enhanced sense of accomplishment and satisfaction

* Better tracking and evaluation of progress

* Increased chances of achieving the desired outcome

Here is a helpful video to help you set SMART goals:

https://bit.ly/SMART-goals-blueprint

CORE CONDITIONING

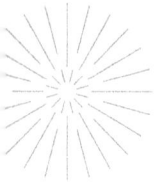

What Is It?

As defined earlier, the **core** is the trunk of your body—from the diaphragm to the pelvic floor—and **conditioning** is how you keep it strong. Note that core conditioning is not about achieving the abdominal "six-pack" of some athletes, models, and other fitness gurus, but rather strengthening the central "cylinder" of your body. This is formed by muscles deep in front and to your sides (transverse abdominus); the deep back muscles (multifidi); your diaphragm, which supports breathing; and your pelvic floor muscles, which support your urinary and genital organs.

spine and spine muscles

diaphragm

multifidus

abdominal wall muscles

transversus abdominis

pelvic floor muscles

PELVIC GURU

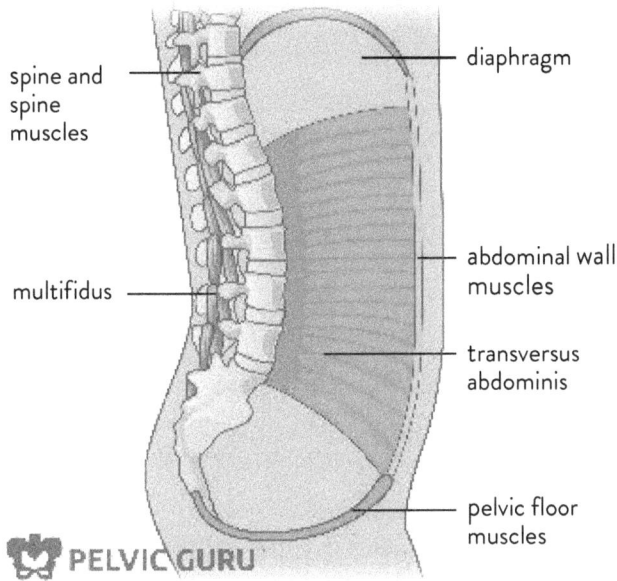

Many people find it helpful to see a visual demonstration of these muscles, instead of merely an image or a description. The following video offers an excellent animation of core muscle anatomy (though it does not include the diaphragm):

https://bit.ly/core-muscle-demo

Why Is It Important?

Your core muscles are critical for supporting your spine and all internal organs below the diaphragm and above the pelvic floor. They also help you maintain good posture. As you can imagine, core strength and postural alignment play a substantial role in how you look, feel, and function.

How Do You Achieve It?

Contrary to popular belief, sit-ups are not the way to strengthen your core. In fact, for those of us at risk for osteoporotic fractures, they are actually dangerous. The way most people do them induces a compression force on the upper-middle bones of your spine (thoracic vertebrae), which can cause a fracture. This is what leads to the hunched backs (kyphosis) we see in so many older people—which you can hopefully prevent by being mindful of your posture and body mechanics during activities.

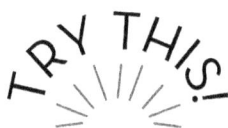

TRY THIS!

The following exercise comes from the work of Sara Meeks, PT (who also contributed Chapter 10 on osteoporosis management). This is another isometric exercise, so as we discussed earlier, it is imperative that you practice *conscious* breathing the entire time.

THE FOOT PRESS EXERCISE

1. Perch or sit forward on the edge of a firm chair, and plant your feet flat on the floor, hip-width apart. Be sure you are wearing non-slip shoes for this exercise, or it may be difficult to gain the traction you need. You can also do this activity while standing.

2. Do at least three sets of *conscious* breathing cycles to ensure you do not hold your breath while doing this isometric.

3. Get into your best postural alignment by using the suggestion "Lengthen – Open – Make space in your chest." Let your chin tuck in and back (retract) and imagine a string or cord pulling the crown of your head toward the ceiling. Note here that the suggestion to "open" is to encourage you to relax the accessory muscles around your neck, shoulders, and chest. These muscles have no role in your postural/core conditioning.

4. As you continue your conscious breathing, slowly and steadily press down into your feet, as if trying to push through heavy, wet cement. At the same time, imagine pressing the crown of your head higher toward the ceiling. **The exaggerated "lengthening" of the spine is key in this exercise.**

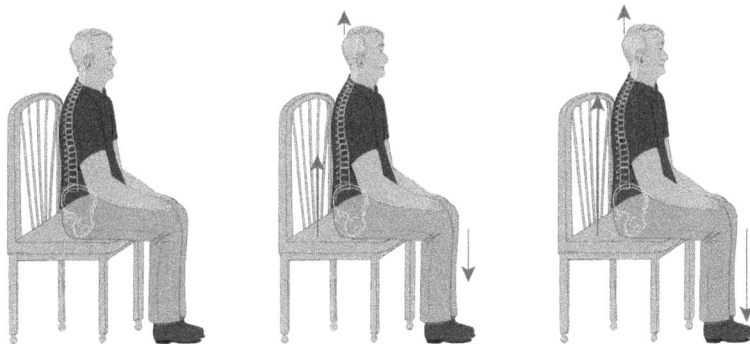

5. Maintain a steady conscious breathing pattern while pressing your feet down into the floor and the crown of your head toward the ceiling until your muscles begin to fatigue.

6. Now, slowly stop pressing but maintain your good postural alignment.

7. Continue to do your conscious breathing. Repeat this activity at least three to four more times, if you're able. Remember, the more sets and repetitions you work into your day, the stronger your core will become, and the better your posture and even endurance!

Finally, I want to remind you that because this is an isometric exercise, burning or shaking, especially in the muscles of your thighs, buttocks, and up your back, is normal and an indicator that you're doing it right.

DIAPHRAGMATIC BREATHING AND CONDITIONING

Remember the diaphragmatic breathing you learned in Chapter 2? Performing these *conscious* breathing exercises is how you condition the diaphragm and your entire breathing apparatus for improved endurance and increased respiratory capacity.

As a refresher, here are the steps once again:

1. Sit or lie in a comfortable, supported position.

2. Close your eyes and begin *consciously* breathing. If you generally breathe through your mouth, **try to breathe in through your nose**. If your breath is high in your chest, try to relax it and strive to let your stomach expand as you inhale ("Balloon Breathing").

3. Place your hands gently on your abdomen, just under your rib cage and slightly to the sides of your trunk. Make sure your chest is relaxed and your shoulders are down (not in a shrugged position).

4. Imagine filling a balloon in your abdomen with air as you inhale. Another image is to imagine smelling your favorite fragrance.

5. Become conscious of your abdomen rising as you breathe in. (This is not meant to be a "deep breath," which would force your chest to rise, but rather a gentle inhalation so you can feel the diaphragm working.)

6. Purse your lips, as if to whistle, as you prepare to exhale. You can also make a hissing sound, like you'd hear from a leaky tire.

7. Time how long you can sustain pursed-lip or leaky-tire breathing. (You can count to yourself or use the second hand of a clock or watch to time yourself.)

8. Although you can exhale using your nose *or* mouth, I encourage you to practice slow, prolonged exhalations through pursed lips. This allows stale or "residual" air to be removed from the corners of the lungs, making more room for energy-giving, oxygenated air when you breathe in again.

   Disclaimer: A device I use and promote is called The Breather by PN Medical. It has variable settings that allow you to resist inhalation and exhalation, which in turn strengthens the diaphragm, back, and abdominal muscles. (Check it out in "My Favorite Things" section at the end of this book.)

PELVIC FLOOR CONDITIONING

Unfortunately for both men and women, we can experience issues with bowel, bladder, and even sexual function when pelvic floor muscles are allowed to stretch, sag, and weaken. But no matter your age, you will benefit from learning how to engage and strengthen those muscles.

You've probably heard of (or even done) Kegel exercises for strengthening your pelvic floor. These are excellent; however, it's imperative that you learn how to do them correctly. I recommend working with a qualified health or fitness professional to achieve this, but the following videos are also helpful:

https://bit.ly/Kegels-for-women
https://bit.ly/Kegels-for-men

I must caution you that many people suggest stopping the flow of urine as an effective way to condition the pelvic area of your core, but this is definitely NOT a recommended, effective, or safe course of action. Kegels are a much better method.

The prior three core-conditioning exercises are the ones I've found to be the simplest and most productive. However, if you'd like to explore more options, there are ample routines online and in books that you might enjoy. Just keep in mind that regardless of which ones you choose, always start with The ABCs (Align–Breathe–Center), progress slowly so that you can stop any activity if it feels unsafe or uncomfortable, and consult with your healthcare provider if you have questions about how or what you've decided to adopt as a practice.

FUNCTIONAL FITNESS

What Is It?

Functional fitness refers to any exercise that is intended to help you perform your daily activities with greater safety, ease, and efficiency, such as the bending, lifting, and reaching you do to manage your self-care, your home, your recreational activities, etc. When you focus on functional fitness, your goal is to foster the strength, flexibility, and endurance to be able to do all of those activities—with energy to spare.

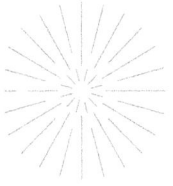

Why Is It Important?

We all want to function independently, yet so many of us either become lazy as we age, or we become bogged down with aches, pains, and conditions that limit our mobility (usually from not being mobile enough!). Being able to perform all the everyday tasks of our lives—and those that are much more fun!—is why functional fitness should be important to everyone.

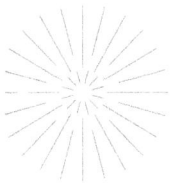

How Do You Achieve It?

Essentially, you want to turn everyday actions into "fitness" activities by mimicking the characteristics of normal, "functional" movements. The two videos below are excellent for seniors in that they utilize a chair; however, they are great for anyone at any age to foster gentle conditioning. In spite of their titles, they work the full body, especially if you integrate your ABCs into them.

https://bit.ly/upper-body-mobility
https://bit.ly/lower-body-mobility

In setting functional fitness goals, here are questions you can ask yourself, then set a SMART goal for each:

* How far do I want to walk?

* How high do I want to reach?

* How heavy is the grandchild I want to lift without straining my back? (I realize children grow at a rapid rate, so their weight isn't stagnant,

but you can work toward lifting their current weight, plus five pounds.)

* How far do I want to hit a golf ball?

* How long into the night do I want to dance?

* How many tennis or pickleball sets do I want to play?

* How much gardening do I want to be able to do?

You get the idea. Functional fitness is the approach to exercise that focuses on the activities that are important for you in your everyday life. What else might you add to the list?

FROM THE GROUND UP

Assessing the activities you want to be able to do is a vital component of improving your ability to age safely, wisely, and well. But there's also something you may not think about, and that's getting down and up from the floor. I hope this will never be the case because of a fall, but there are several scenarios that could have you on the floor intentionally: doing one of the activities in this book that has the option of lying down, finding a dropped contact lens, crawling around with grandchildren . . . you get the idea. And once the activity is done, you've got to get yourself up!

Because this can be difficult for some people, let's look at a step by step of the safest way to condition yourself for that kind of functional necessity.

1. Place a sturdy chair in front of you (seat facing you) with a pillow on the floor in front of it, such that you can stand about one foot away from the seat of the chair.

2. Align, Breathe, and Center yourself.

3. Bend at the waist and place your hands on both sides of the seat of the chair. You will still be standing, but in an inverted V position.

4. Now, *slowly* lower yourself down, one knee at a time, onto the cushion. You may bend your arms and rest your elbows on the seat of the chair as you try to get down onto both knees.

5. From here, if you are able, lie down on the floor. Take some time to breathe and relax.

6. When you're ready to get back up, bend your knees with your feet on the floor.

7. Roll onto your stronger side, if you have one.

8. Push yourself up to a side-sitting position.

9. Stop. Breathe.

10. Next, *slowly* bring yourself into a hands and knees position.

11. Gently move toward the firm seat you are going to use to help you get up from the ground. (It may or may not be the one you started with.)

12. Place your forearms on the seat, then raise your stronger leg up in front of you, or as close as possible. This is called a half-kneeling position.

13. Stop and breathe again.

14. From here, push yourself up to standing with both arms now straight on the seat of the chair supporting you.

15. Stop and breathe yet again.

16. Finally, in *S-l-o-w–M-o-t-i-o-n*, turn yourself around so you can sit down in the chair.

For an excellent demonstration of both getting onto the floor and up from it, please watch the following video:

https://bit.ly/down-to-and-up-from-floor

Remember to prepare yourself by taking a moment to mentally practice the skill and have your focus strictly on the activity you are about to begin. Secondly, do the entire sequence in *S-l-o-w–M-o-t-i-o-n* to ensure you can stop or reverse the action in case you have some discomfort or feel you don't have complete control over it. If pain or weakness limits your ability to do the full sequence, repeat the part of it you can do comfortably and safely. This will allow you to develop the strength, flexibility, and skill you need to perform the entire activity—and to continue on your path of being "functionally fit."

TIPS FOR GETTING THE MOST FROM YOUR FITNESS ROUTINE

Before you undertake a fitness program, or any of the activities in this book, here are some tips for achieving maximum benefits with minimum risk of pain or injury.

1. Set SMART Goals to identify exactly what you want to improve, and how you want to look, feel, and function.

2. Begin each activity with The ABC Mind-Body System: Align – Breathe – Center.

3. Do each exercise *s-l-o-w-l-y.* This will give you more control and help you develop strength, balance, and control. It will also help you master new movements or exercises. (I know I said this is not an "exercise" book, but you may be inspired to do them.)

4. Use a full-length mirror and music to make your activities more effective and fun! The mirror will give you feedback about your posture and technique, while the music will stimulate your desire to move.

5. Increase your flexibility, strength, balance, coordination, and endurance by doing "freestyle movements," meaning movements done in all directions, like in ballet or modern dance. Continuous, rhythmic body motion improves the ability of your body to use oxygen (aerobic capacity) and improve your general condition.

6. Keep a record of your progress. This can be highly motivating and helpful for planning the progression of your program. For example, if you can currently sit and stand from your chair three times without stopping, can you increase that number to five, and then to ten?

7. To avoid injury, always listen to your body and let it be your guide. Make safe movement your priority. Learn the difference between pain that indicates something is not beneficial and perhaps even harmful to your body, versus the discomfort that may come during stretching or strengthening activities.

8. Share your program and progress with family and friends. You may even motivate them to get up and move with you.

9. Now, get up and move, breathe, and enjoy!

Chapter 7

The Gift of Balance:
A Blueprint for Staying Steady
on Your Feet and Preventing Falls

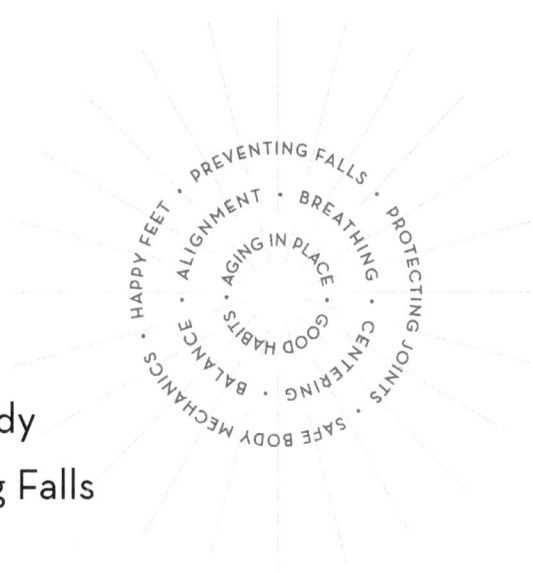

W e've all heard the stories or experienced it in our own families—or maybe it's even happened to you: "After my mother / father / grandmother / grandfather fell and broke their hip, they were never the same. They really declined after that."

Yikes!

That bleak prospect is enough to scare anyone into wanting to maintain good balance!

The problem is, balance issues tend to sneak up on us gradually as we age, especially if we aren't doing the kinds of functional exercise and activity I've taught you thus far in the book, or we begin spending more time sitting than being active. Shock may come when one day you squat to get something from a lower shelf in the grocery store and realize your hips and knees are so weak that you can't use them to get back to a standing position, at least not without pushing yourself up from the floor with your hands or holding on to something or someone for leverage. Or perhaps you simply catch your foot on a lip in the sidewalk and find out the hard way that you can't regain your balance the way you used to.

Scenarios abound for how people slowly find themselves not as steady or strong on their feet as they once were, yet instead of thoughtfully analyzing the cause(s) and making changes that could turn that situation around, they simply chalk it up to aging. Well, I am here to tell you, after five decades as a practicing physical therapist, that this is one of the most deceptive untruths we've been led to believe—and we're going to spend this chapter doing something about that!

Much of the information in this chapter is thanks to my friend Cate Reade, MS, RD, exercise physiologist, corrective exercise specialist, and registered dietician. Cate has worked with older adults for over a decade and has heard countless stories of how balance and mobility issues have limited their activities and lives. She is also the inventor and distributor of MoveMor, a resistance exercise device for foot, ankle, and general leg conditioning. More on this fabulous device later in the chapter.

Further contributions to this chapter come from Dr. Rein Tideiksaar, PhD, PA, a friend and renowned researcher in the field of preventing falls. You will find numerous books, articles, and videos by him online, and I highly recommend you check them out.

Combining these excellent contributors' content into one comprehensive chapter, we will focus on the three key factors of keeping you in balance: 1) **visual, auditory, and kinetic health;** 2) **the strength and flexibility of joints;** and 3) **wearing the proper shoes,** all of which will aid in the overarching goal of **preventing falls.**

To get started, let's explore the topic of **balance** as the foundation for keeping you confident and steady on your feet, so that the fear of falling no longer dampens your jig as you move into your golden years.

What Is It?

Balance is essentially your ability to keep your body's center of gravity (COG) over your base of support (BOS). You've already learned about COG in the section on Centering in Chapter 2, and about BOS in Chapter 4 in the discussion of the Basic Moves. Although it's not demonstrated here, your COG and BOS will change depending on your position and activity

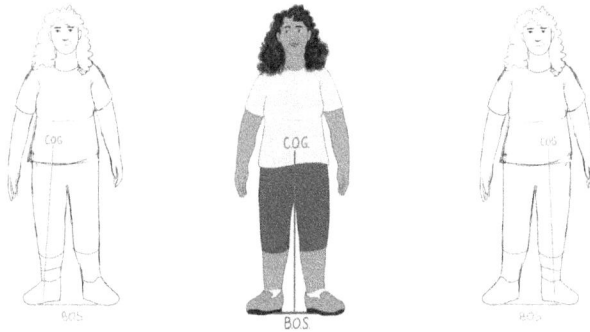

"Dynamic" balance is your ability to maintain your COG over your BOS **when you are in motion.** Think of the movements a person makes balancing on a tightrope. They constantly move their body parts to keep their balance. Your body does the same when you are walking, especially when you encounter a curb or uneven surface. When your arms are swinging naturally as you stride, or your core goes into extra support mode if you trip or get off balance, your COG is constantly adjusting to stay over your BOS. **This is how your body prevents itself from falling.**

When you were practicing The Basic Moves for the first time, did you notice it was easier to be stable when you had a larger base of support? A great example is to imagine the difference in stability between a cone placed with the large side down versus trying to get it to stand on its pointy end. The same is true when you strive to keep your balance while standing with your legs tightly together and performing actions with your upper body, versus standing with your legs farther apart and doing those same actions. Widening your BOS—not to an exaggerated width but to a natural distance—allows you to better maintain your COG, which in turn enables better balance and stability. You would experience the same marked difference if you compared standing on one leg to standing with your legs apart in a solid stance (but don't try it if you already have balance issues—**remember, safety first!**).

Why Is It Important?

It goes without saying that by helping you minimize slips, trips, and stumbles that can injure or land you in the hospital, balance is the primary reason you remain on your feet and off the ground. It is also what allows you to sit, stand, and perform everyday tasks safely. But having good balance goes beyond the physical. It is psychological as well.

If you have poor balance, it can not only negatively affect your confidence, but it can cause depression. You may have a decreased desire to go anywhere that would challenge your balance, particularly if you are self-conscious about using a walking aid, like a cane or walker. It may also reduce your willingness to socialize, which science has proven to be a key element in our ability to age mentally and physically well. After all, humans are designed to be social beings and to need each other!

Finally, if you carry a persistent fear of falling because you don't trust your balance, that fear has a substantial impact on how your body responds mentally and physically to situations that potentially challenge your balance. Remember the elderly woman with a hip fracture in Chapter 5, in the segment on Self-Talk, who said "I can't" so many times that she made her body believe she couldn't walk, not even with help, after her hip surgery? Yet simply saying "I'll try" *one time* transformed her willingness and ability to get up and walk in an instant! Her fear was disabling her, and if it may be disabling you too, keep reading.

I don't have to tell you that the above concerns are potentially detrimental for your physical as well as mental health. But the good news is that with a little effort, you can build your confidence simply by understanding and developing your balance skills—which we will do shortly. But before we jump to action steps, let's take a moment to absorb some encouraging words from Cate:

> "No matter what your current condition, take a deep breath and know that you can restore your balance, strength, and confidence. Given the right stimulation, you can improve your physical function to move steadier, stronger, and faster. Your confidence and energy levels will rise with greater positivity so that you can live your independent best."

Sound good? Let's continue!

THE PHYSICAL COMPONENTS OF BALANCE

Balance relies on information flowing to and from three main systems in your brain. They are called "sensory" systems because they pick up information from your eyes (**visual**), your ears (**vestibular**), and the nerves in your joints and muscles (**proprioceptive**).

Moving safely and efficiently depends on your brain's ability to gather and interpret information from all three systems. Obviously, damage to or dysfunction in any of these systems will present a challenge to your balance.

Visual System

Whether you are in an unfamiliar place like a busy airport, campground, or mall; an open outdoor space like a beach or garden; or a completely familiar space, such as your home or local grocery store, your eyes tell your brain where your body is relative to the environment. So it stands to reason that as our eyesight weakens, so does the quality of our sensory input.

This is why it's vital for you to have regular vision checkups. And for those of you who think glasses make you less handsome or attractive, there are dozens of flattering frames available that will not only suit your face and coloring, but can also enhance your appearance. So have fun picking out and wearing glasses to improve not only how you see, but how you look. They may even become your favorite accessory!

Vestibular System

Do you know that much of your balance depends on your ears? This is because structures within the ears sense the position and movement of your head, which means that your inner ear can be thought of as both a level and accelerometer (an instrument for detecting and measuring vibrations).

Semicircular canals within the ear contain fluid and tiny hair cells, and as you nod up and down, move left or right, or tilt your head to the side, that fluid moves. Those tiny hair cells sense the speed and direction of your head's movement and communicate that information to your brain, which then adjusts your posture for improved balance.

Unfortunately, by age 70, it's typical to have lost 40 percent of these sensory-detecting hair cells. Exposure to loud music, wearing headsets with the volume too high, or working in a noisy environment are usually the culprits of damaging those delicate cells over time. This is why it is essential to have your ears and hearing checked annually. While you may not be able to reverse the damage (though promising natural remedies and technologies are discovered all the time), it may be worth looking into a hearing device. Likewise, if you suffer from tinnitus, you should seek a remedy as quickly as possible. As with vision, research has shown a relationship between hearing and balance, so enhancing your ability to hear can aid in your ability to maintain good balance.

Proprioceptive System

Proprioception, also known as kinesthesia, refers to your body's ability to sense how it is moving, both how fast and in what direction. This incredible sensory awareness is made possible by proprioceptors—specialized nerve cells that live in and around your joints, and within ligaments, joint capsules, tendons, muscles, and connective tissues. They not only sense and send signals to the brain about joint position and motion, but they sense the muscle force involved in movement as well.

To put this ability into context, it is similar to having a conversation with a friend on a cell phone with either a weak or a strong connection. If your friend calls for advice and you can only hear every third word she says, you won't be able to advise her very well; it's inevitable that important information will be left out. But with a stronger connection, where you can hear every word, you receive an uninterrupted flow of information and feel much more confident in offering guidance.

In the same way, poor sensory input results in a brain that doesn't have enough information to properly advise the body on how to stay upright and balanced. In other words, without proprioception, you would be unable to move without thinking about each subsequent action, such as walking without having to think about where to place your foot next.

Proprioception also enables you to do things like touch your finger to your nose with your eyes closed. This is because nerve endings are sensing what you're doing and how you're doing it, without being dependent on your eyes or ears.

As you might imagine, proprioception is a prerequisite for balance and safe, effective movement. As part of your body's unconscious self-awareness system, it detects where your body parts are and what they are doing, which enables you to move freely without having to consciously control your movements. And when you *do* want to control your movements, such as when you are learning a new skill, proprioception aids in allowing that as well.

OTHER CAUSES OF BALANCE ISSUES

Several diseases and conditions can cause abnormalities of balance, including diabetes, Parkinson's, stroke, arthritis, and even low blood pressure. In some people, balance difficulties may be an early indication of an underlying disease condition yet to surface. However, diseases are not the only reason for balance loss. A history of injuries, such as concussions, ear infections, or serious sprains or fractures, may contribute to a loss of balance over time. Lastly, both prescription and over-the-counter medications can be detrimental to your balance, so it is vital that you be aware of these side effects and try to find healthier options than drugs. Be sure to work with a healthcare professional who is versed in uncovering root causes of balance issues, rather than masking the issue with a potentially harmful pharmaceutical.

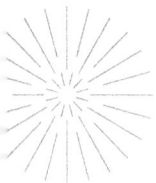

How Do You Achieve Better Balance?

I know, having all of this basic science knowledge is great, and hopefully you now have a better understanding of the components that make balance possible and what can negatively affect it. But the question everyone wants answered is: How do I achieve and maintain good balance?

Well, it begins with the **three sensory systems** we just discussed and ensuring each of them is operating at the highest level possible for you. You may want to set a baseline by visiting an opthamalogist, an audiologist, and a physical therapist. These professionals can provide the appropriate tests to ensure that your **visual, vestibular**, and **proprioceptive** systems are functioning efficiently—and where you might need some assistance to boost them.

The guidance that follows is meant to provide helpful solutions to balance issues, in combination with clinical testing and recommendations, such as eyeglasses, treatments for eye conditions, hearing devices, assistive devices, etc. Taken together, the hope is that you can improve your balance, prevent falls, and improve your confidence and sense of well-being.

AGE-RELATED VISUAL CHANGES AND HELPFUL SOLUTIONS

Many people experience visual issues with age, but this challenge does *not* have to bring you down or limit your capacity to enjoy life. Yes, there are extreme cases, such as advanced macular degeneration or progressive blindness, but the majority of visual changes are not at all difficult to manage; you simply need some tips! I have highlighted below the most common changes people experience and offer helpful solutions for each.

Visual Change: An inability of the eyes to adjust to brighter light.

Helpful Solutions

- Be aware that when you are moving from a dimly lit room into bright lighting, you may experience temporary blindness until your eyes adjust to the dramatic change, so give yourself those extra seconds to regain clear vision before taking more steps.

- Avoid abrupt lighting changes indoors by using dimmer switches to turn up lights.

- Be extra cautious when walking outside on sunny days, particularly when the glare is intense. Be sure your eyes are adjusted before moving from place to place.

Visual Change: A loss of dark adaptation, particularly when moving from outdoors to indoors, from a bright room to a dark room, or moving about at night.

Helpful Solutions

- As when moving from dim to bright light, be aware that moving from bright to dim light or darkness can cause temporary blindness until your eyes adjust, so again, give yourself those extra seconds to adapt.

- Make sure that commonly used areas of your home (stairways, hallways, bedrooms, and bathrooms) have sufficient light. Install bright lighting in all rooms to avoid tripping over objects that are not easy to see.

- Try smart lights. Whether they are triggered by motion or come on at pre-specified times, smart lights turn on without having to use switches.

- Use nightlights to make navigation in the dark easier and safer, especially if you get up frequently during the night to use the bathroom.

- Outside, consider installing motion-sensor flood lights or increasing lighting on exterior pathways, porches, and doorways.

Visual Change: A greater sensitivity to glare. Common sources of glare include sunlight shining through windows and reflecting off glossy floors, and bright light from unshielded light fixtures directed toward your eye. Glare is troublesome because it hides potential fall hazards.

Helpful Solutions

- Avoid lighting glare by repositioning lamps or use lampshades.
- Avoid floor glare by using carpets and nonslip floor finishes that diffuse rather than reflect.

Visual Change: Cataracts—a gradual clouding of the lens that affects mobility and balance by reducing the perception of the edges of steps and sidewalks, as well as altering depth perception of the ground.

Helpful Solution

- Visit your ophthalmologist to discuss cataract surgery. Though all surgeries carry risk, this is a common procedure, and most people regain substantial vision by having the cataracts removed. Lens replacement is often an option during cataract surgery as well, which can correct visual impairment in some circumstances.

AMPLIFYING AND SUPPORTING HEARING FOR OVERALL HEALTH

While hearing is connected to your balance, and that reason alone is enough to care about the health of your ears, there are three additional reasons as well. According to a 2020 *Lancet* commission report:

1. Hearing loss leads to a greater chance of developing dementia. This is because hearing loss causes the brain to work harder, forcing it to strain to hear and fill in the gaps. As you might imagine, this comes at the expense of other thinking and memory systems.

2. Hearing loss causes an aging brain to shrink more quickly.

3. Hearing loss leads people to be less socially engaged, which is hugely important to remaining intellectually stimulated. If you can't hear very well, you may not go out as much, so the brain is less engaged and active.

I share this with you not to scare or discourage you, but rather to encourage and empower you to ensure hearing loss isn't damaging you in more ways than you may realize. I, myself, have diminished hearing, which involves a decreased ability to hear higher pitches. I was reluctant to explore getting hearing aids because of unfavorable stories I'd heard about them making *all* sounds louder, which was an annoying feature in older units. I was happy to discover, however, that today's models are customized to an individual's particular hearing loss. In my case, the devices round out my ability to hear the higher ranges of sound I was losing, which has been wonderful for listening to music again, among other things.

I hope that if you're experiencing hearing loss of any kind, you won't be hesitant or fearful of having your ears checked by an audiologist—and that if you need it, you'll feel empowered in considering a personalized hearing aid solution. Your brain, balance, and social life can only benefit!

For a detailed demonstration on ear anatomy and function,
I recommend the following video:
https://bit.ly/ear-anatomy-and-function

SUPPORTING THE PROPRIOCEPTIVE SYSTEM BY IMPROVING JOINT STRENGTH AND FLEXIBILITY

You already know that proprioception—or kinesthesia—refers to your body's ability to sense how it is moving, both how fast and in what direction, via sensory nerves that live in and around joints, ligaments, tendons, muscles, and connective tissues. In this section, we are going to focus on improving specific ones: those that reside in the feet and ankles.

Not only do your feet and ankles provide the physical foundation for balance when you are standing, they also contain sensors that are critical for your ability to sense where your body is. (Up to 70 percent of the sensory input for balance comes from your joints!) The strength, flexibility, and proprioceptors in your feet and ankles enable them to sense and respond as your Center of Gravity (COG) shifts over your Base of Support (BOS) while standing and walking. In simple terms, all of these factors allow you to be in balance.

Being farthest from the heart and blood flow, research shows that your ankles are the first joints to decline, making them prone to stiffness and immobility. As your base, this has rippling effects up and down the kinetic chain. In other words, with a weak, unstable base, the rest of the body compensates to make movement happen.

The most common ranges of motion lost is dorsiflexion (the lifting of the foot at the ankle), making it difficult to raise your foot as you step forward. Your foot might actually point down into plantarflexion, a frequent cause of falls while walking or navigating stairs. One of the consequences is that it may lead to your feet becoming unstable as the arches weaken and the foot flattens. To compensate, your feet might turn outward, causing your knees to roll inward, your hips to shift down, your pelvis to tilt forward, and your shoulders to hunch. These misalignments result in tightness, stress, and strain that increases the wear and tear on joints. What follows is dysfunction, degeneration, inflammation, and pain throughout your body. Ankle stiffness is an often overlooked reason for pain in the foot, ankle, knee, hip, back, shoulder, and even neck.

The solution?

Fix your foundation!

By simply moving your ankles in all directions, through all three planes of motion (exercises to follow), you can condition those hard-to-reach lower leg and foot muscles to create a strong, flexible, and stable base of support for better balance. You and your body are resilient, and yes! You *can* improve your balance and mobility with foot and ankle conditioning because it can:

* Strengthen feet and lower legs
* Support foot arches
* Increase foot mobility, stability, and circulation
* Help improve body alignment
* Improve walking speed and gait pattern
* Improve proprioception
* Strengthen neuromuscular connections
* Support enhanced balance reflexes
* Help restore functional independence
* Build confidence and fall resilience

By training your feet and ankles through a full, pain-free range of motion, you will be able to depend on them to be more agile and give you better balance in your everyday life—hopefully saving yourself from falls. But before we get to preventing falls, let's spend a few minutes giving attention to the marvel that is your feet!

APPRECIATING YOUR WONDROUS FEET!

1. Take a moment to notice your feet, toes, and ankles. Move them around a little. Now ask yourself the following questions:

    - Have they been your friends over the years?
    - Do they hurt?
    - Are they stiff and swollen?
    - Have they ever received any professional care, such as a podiatrist visit or a pedicure?
    - Do you have positive feelings about them, or have you considered them unattractive and something to be hidden?
    - Have you spent years cramming them into ill-fitting, pointy-toed shoes?

2. Now, if you're able to do it safely, stand barefoot on the floor. Look down at your feet and s-l-o-w-l-y shift your weight forward and back, and side to side. Notice how the little muscles in your feet move as they work to help you balance. Take a few moments to appreciate the large role they play in helping you stay upright and avoid a fall.

GIVE YOUR FEET SOME LOVE!

When you tend to your feet, they will be more able to do their job. (We will talk more about this topic in the next chapter: Healthy Feet Are Happy Feet.) But for now, here are a few tips for giving your feet some love:

- Make sure the skin of your feet and around your toes is in good condition and that you tend to any potential issues. If you can manage a monthly pedicure, skin care is typically part of the appointment. This can help you to avoid cracked skin, sores, and overgrown or sharp nails that can cause you problems.

- While dressing and bathing, strive to maintain the range of motion of your toes, mid-foot, and ankle joint. If you can't reach your toes to clean and stimulate the skin between them, there are long-handled devices with brushes and terrycloth ends to make the job easier. (See page 176 in the My Favorite Things section.)

- Stimulate the soles of your feet by using a cloth or towel, or by standing on a textured mat or carpet. This wakes them up and increases sensitivity—which enhances proprioception. (Do use caution if you have neuropathy or decreased sensation in your feet, as you don't want to risk a fall, skin irritation, or a sore.)

WATCH THEM WORK!

Becoming mindful, developing awareness, and learning to s-l-o-w d-o-w-n are first steps to achieving better balance. The following weight-shifting sequence is designed to increase your awareness and appreciation of how involved your feet are with balance. The moves may seem too slow and simple, but trust me, they are effective (and they can help you develop the proprioceptive awareness described earlier). If you are able to be safe, close your eyes during this activity.

Before you start, remember to stand with good **Alignment** and do *conscious* **Breathing** as you perform each activity, then return to **Center** before changing directions.

1. Shift your weight s-l-o-w-l-y from your center of gravity toward your toes. Notice how your toes curl and your feet press down as they work to keep you from tipping forward. Then return to your Center, squarely in the middle of both feet.

2. Now, shift your weight s-l-o-w-l-y back toward your heels. Notice how your toes and feet want to pull up? Return to your Center, as above.

3. Do a s-l-o-w weight shift toward the right side of both feet. Return to your Center, as above. (If one side is stronger than the other, go to that side first.) Then do the opposite side. Feel yourself get taller as your weight is shifted onto one side.

4. Keeping that nice, tall Alignment, s-l-o-w-l-y turn/twist your upper body to one side. Do you feel how the muscles in your feet are responding? That's what you want to notice. Return to your Center. Repeat the turn/twist toward the other side.

Your goal is to start appreciating how hard your feet work to keep you upright. My hope is that this understanding and appreciation will be the motivation you need to give your feet the love and respect they deserve. Your feet will thank you and be able to work and serve you well through the rest of your life.

FOOT AND ANKLE CONDITIONING FOR BETTER BALANCE

Besides sending your feet some love, the following exercises will help them develop the strength and flexibility they need to serve you.

First, you'll stretch your ankle to allow for more range of motion. You can use a wall or sturdy countertop for support.

1. Align – Breathe – Center.

2. Keeping your heel flat on the floor, s-l-o-w-l-y press forward from your hips until you feel a pull in the back of your calf. Now stop.

3. Inhale, then press forward as you exhale.

4. Do this at least 3 to 5 times until you feel you have achieved the maximum stretch.

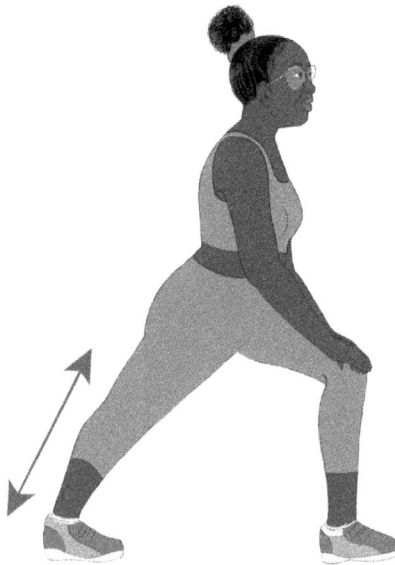

You are now ready to do a few exercises for foot and ankle conditioning. Many more exist than those that follow, but I find these to
be great for beginners.

- Most exercise can be performed while lying down or sitting,
  and with or without elastic band resistance. Later, you can
  add resistance with a device or your own body weight as
  you do them in a standing position.

- Perform these exercises through your fullest pain-free range
  of motion.

- If a movement causes pain, it is your body's signal to stop.
  Make the movement smaller, slower, or stop altogether.

- Try to do activities in "sets" (3 on average) of 5 to 10
  "repetitions" (reps) scattered throughout your day. You can
  modify these numbers depending on your strength and
  endurance. Both should increase as you progress.

- Remember, we are *transforming* the ways you move through
  life, so these activities are best integrated throughout your
  regular day.

Ready?

1. Align – Breathe – Center.

2. Decide if you want to perform the activity in a sitting or
   lying position, based on your comfort and safety.

3. If you have a stronger side, start with that one. I call it your
   "teacher" side.

FOOT AND TOE LIFTS (ANKLE DORSIFLEXION)

1. Bend your feet and toes upward (ankle dorsiflexion).

2. Hold them up for several seconds, then relax them.

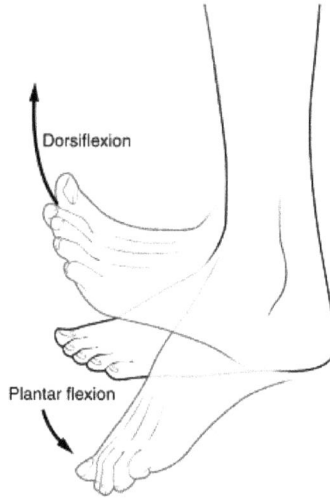

HEEL LIFTS

1. Point your foot and toes down and raise your heels up as high as possible (plantarflexion). If you are seated with your feet on the floor, you'll be pressing down on the balls of your feet.

2. Hold for several seconds, then relax.

FOOT AND ANKLE CIRCLES

1. Make *s-l-o-w*, *large* circles with your feet and ankles. (Imagine you have a paint brush at the tip of your big toe and are trying to draw the largest circle possible.)

2. Now repeat in the opposite direction.

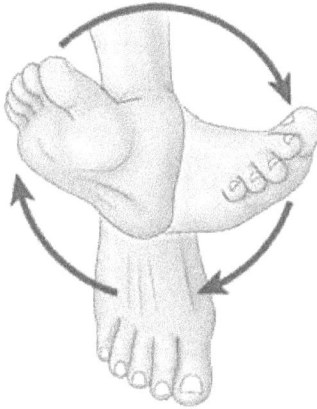

OVER-THE-HILL EXERCISE

This exercise came from a sports therapy expert. For this one, start in a seated position. As your foot and ankle become stronger and more flexible, you'll be able to progress to doing it while standing with support.

Note: You will know you are a foot and ankle hero if you can eventually do this exercise without needing support. However, this might not be safe or practical if your foot strength and mobility is limited.

1. With your feet and ankles warmed up from the first three exercises, sit forward on a supportive seat.

2. Align – Breathe – Center.

3. Raise your heels up (Heel Lift) and point your toes down
    into the floor. We'll call it the "Toe-Stand" position. (If you
    are standing, you will be on the balls of your feet, not on
    downward pointed toes—unless you are a trained ballet
    dancer!)

4. Keeping your heels up, s-l-o-w-l-y roll your feet and ankles to
    one side, choosing your stronger or easier side first. You are
    striving to be on the outer border of one foot and the inner
    border of the other foot. In other words, your feet will not
    be flat on the ground.

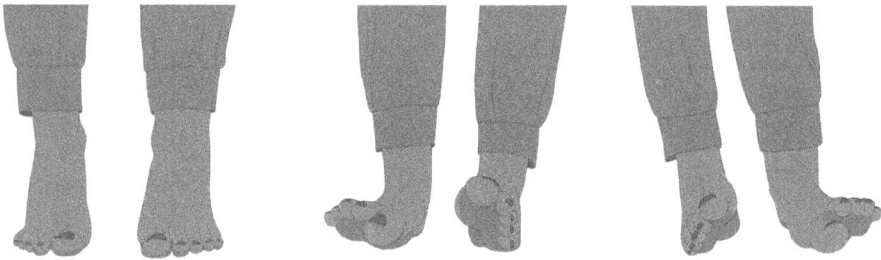

5. S-l-o-w-l-y roll your feet and ankles back up to the Toe-Stand
    position.

6. S-l-o-w-l-y roll your feet and ankles over to the other side.

7. Return to the Toe-Stand position.

8. Repeat 3–5 times, rest, then repeat again, for three total
    sets of 8 if you're able.

With all of the above exercises, what's great is that you can perform them
throughout your day. My recommendation is to get into the habit of doing
them while sitting and watching TV, when you're at the computer, or while

waiting for an appointment. Consistency is key, so if you can integrate these into your daily routine, you should feel a steady increase in foot and ankle strength and flexibility.

If you're interested in or ready for advanced foot and ankle conditioning, I recommend this video:

https://bit.ly/foot-and-ankle-advanced

While these exercises may not be appropriate or even possible for you, you may enjoy watching them as inspiration.

As a final note, if you are experiencing one or more of the following balance issues, I recommend you visit your healthcare professional to explore what kinds of protocols may improve proprioception in your feet and ankles, or if there might be a more serious underlying problem:

* Feeling unsteady when rising from a chair, bed, or toilet.

* Needing to hold on to walls or furniture for support, or staggering from side to side when walking and turning, especially in the dark or under conditions of dim lighting. (This can also indicate visual problems.)

* A sensation of dizziness, lightheadedness, or vertigo (a whirling or spinning movement).

Whether or not these symptoms appear and disappear over short time periods, or last for a longer period, any symptom is your body's way of letting you know something is awry within. By determining the root cause as soon as possible, you can reverse or mitigate most symptoms by giving the body what it needs, so don't accept these kinds of symptoms as simply "aging"— you are meant to thrive in your golden years!

PROGRESSIVE RESISTANCE TRAINING

When you are ready for a greater challenge, you can add varied exercises and/ or some light elastic resistance bands or tubing to see greater improvements in less time. Resistance training through a full range of motion is a highly effective way to improve joint mobility and stability, which are both necessary for safe, efficient movement.

While a single band or tube is helpful, it can take a lot of time and energy to reconfigure yourself and the band for exercising your feet, ankles, knees, and hips. Ankles in particular are notoriously difficult to exercise. So in place of bands and/or tubes, I highly recommend Cate's Movemor Mobility Trainer. It's a frictionless board with variable resistance options for exercising the feet, ankles, and lower extremities beyond what you can do with ordinary resistance bands. Its benefits are backed by research, and it is a simple way for older adults across the continuum of care to improve balance, strength, and mobility in as little as ten minutes per week. We shamelessly promote it at Thera-Fitness!

Visit the MoveMor website to learn more, read testimonials,
and see demonstrations of it in action:
https://www.movemor.com/

FINDING YOUR "SOLE MATE"

Now that you are tuned in to your feet, and you know how to wake them up and get them strong and flexible for balance and walking, it's time to talk about finding the right shoes with the correct fit for you. What follows are guidelines for purchasing shoes that will be your sole mates, not "sole hates"!

* **Determine the arch of your foot.** One way to figure it out is to look at your footprint when you walk with bare feet, perhaps around a pool or on the beach. If you see a bear print, you are flat footed. If you see the heel, a sliver on the outer border of the foot, the ball, and toes, you have a normal foot with a medium arch. If you see only the heel, ball, and toes in the footprint, you have a high arch.

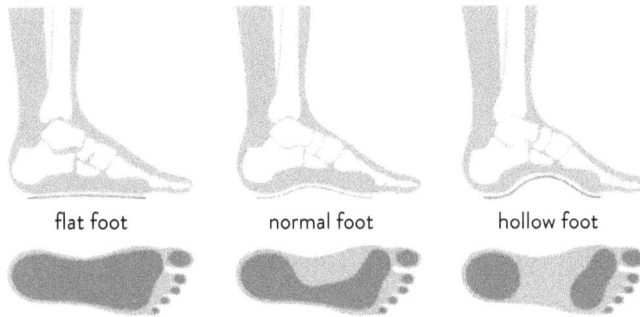

| flat foot | normal foot | hollow foot |

* **Always purchase shoes later in the day.** After you have exercised or been on your feet throughout the day, they are generally more swollen, tired, and sensitive; therefore, you will more easily sense whether the shoe feels comfortable.

* For length, you want approximately a **1/2" of space between the end of your big toe and the end of the shoe**—or half a thumb width to a thumb width when you are standing in it. (Ask the salesperson to check it for you if you cannot reach your toes while standing. Another reason to do your stretching exercises!)

* For width, **make an index card aid.** Get a 3x5 index card (or a larger card if you have big and/or flat feet) and a blank piece of paper. Lay the paper on a flat (not carpeted) surface and stand on it. Mark (or

have someone mark for you) the most inner (medial) aspect of the big toe joint and the most outer (lateral) aspect of the joint behind the little toe. Step off the paper, then place the index card between these two points and mark. Carry this card with you when you purchase shoes, ensuring these two marks fit within the widest portion of the shoe up to a half-inch discrepancy.

✳ **If you have high- or low-arch (flat) feet, get familiar with the "last" of a shoe,** which is the mold or form around which it is built. Shoes typically have a straight, curved, or semi-curved last. If you look at the bottom of your shoe and cannot determine if it is a right or a left shoe, that is a straight last. A curved last will almost look like the letter C. A semi-curved last falls in between. **The high-arch foot typically prefers a curved-last shoe,** which provides better shock absorption. **A flat foot typically prefers straight-last shoes** (also called motion-control shoes), as flat feet will fatigue much faster and are prone to leg cramps as well as general foot and even back pain.

✳ **Don't think that because a shoe is your *usual size* it is the right fit**—the length of the arch of the shoe may not line up with the arch of your foot, and different brands and styles fit differently. (My father used to fit shoes, so I learned that lesson well!)

✳ New shoes **should feel comfortable from the moment you put them on**—if they aren't comfortable when you are seated, imagine how they will feel when you try standing and walking in them. And don't plan on "breaking them in." They will break your foot in first!

✳ Check for correct fit by **standing with your full weight** on your feet. The widest part of the shoe and the widest part of your foot should be aligned. If it's not, you need to try another style or size. If the shoe doesn't fit right, it isn't the right shoe for you.

* If you have an **unusual foot shape or condition,** seek out a pedorthotist —someone who can recommend an appropriate shoe or create a shoe insert or modification to meet your specific needs. www.pedorthics.org

As a last note, supportive shoes with nonskid soles will provide greater safety, as will keeping your shoes in good repair, including replacing the heels if they are worn down, especially if they wear out on an angle or unevenly.

SELF-ASSESSMENT OF FALL RISK FROM DR. REIN

1. Have you fallen one or more times in the past three months?

    Yes____ No____

    Many falls don't "just happen" but are caused by underlying health conditions and/or environmental hazards in the home.

2) Have you stumbled, slipped, or tripped two or more times in the past several weeks?

    Yes____ No____

    This may indicate a problem with walking or seeing correctly.

3) Do you often feel unsteady or lose your balance?

    Yes____ No____

    This may be an early indication of a medical condition that requires looking into.

4) Have you noticed a change in vision?

    Yes____ No____

    Seeing correctly is important in avoiding trips and slips and detecting hazards and objects in one's path.

5) Do you have difficulty walking? Do you sometimes hold on to furniture or walls for support?

    Yes_____ No_____

This may indicate a problem with the nervous system or weak leg muscles.

6) Do you have difficulty getting up from a toilet, chair, or sofa? Difficulty getting in or out of showers or bathtubs? Difficulty walking up/down steps and stairways?

    Yes_____ No_____

This may be a sign of weak muscles or other medical conditions.

7) Do you take several medications daily?

    Yes_____ No_____

Some medications can cause dizziness, drowsiness, and balance problems.

8) Have you noticed a decline in your memory? Easily confused? Feeling depressed?

    Yes_____ No_____

Difficulty with memory or thinking clearly can interfere with safe mobility.

9) Do you exercise regularly?

    Yes_____ No_____

Lack of exercise or inactivity can result in weakened muscles, lack of flexibility, and poor balance.

If you answered yes to one or more of these (except for number 9), do seek the guidance of an appropriate healthcare professional.

STAYING STEADY ON YOUR FEET:
A FEW FINAL TIPS

This chapter has been focused on several elements that create a blueprint for preventing the dreaded fall, and because I know this is a widespread fear so many older people harbor, I hope the useful tools that Cate, Dr. Rein, and I have included have helped to calm that fear for you.

In this final section, I want to offer some further encouragement.

First, if you have a fear of falling, I want to remind you of the "self-talk" strategy we discussed in Chapter 5. When confronted with that fear, say out loud or to yourself, "I am tall, strong, and confident," or "I am going to control you, fear. You're not going to control me!" I've seen these phrases work for many people. Try it yourself!

Second, remember there are simple ways to avoid falls that involve only being a little extra mindful or taking a single action step:

* At home, clear pathways of cords, pet toys, or other objects you may unwittingly trip over.

* Clean eyeglasses often to improve visibility.

* When walking outside or being out and about, be mindful of uneven sidewalks, curbs, speed bumps in parking lots, and lips in door jambs when entering shops. It's always better to slow down and be aware of your surroundings than to rush or be too absorbed in thought or conversation to notice potential hazards.

* Use an assistive device, if needed, and carry/use it with "panache"! Although you may resist it, it may be a good idea for you to use a cane or walker. It doesn't mean you will need it forever; in fact, it is my hope that by following the advice and performing the activities in this book, your need for an assistive device will be temporary. Whether

you need it to give you more confidence while you improve your strength and flexibility, or while you heal from an injury or surgery— or even because of an ongoing physical challenge—there are many different devices to suit your needs. An evaluation by a physical or occupational therapist will help you decide on the one most appropriate for your situation.

* Finally, don't be afraid to ask for the arm of a companion, or even a friendly stranger if you'd feel—or actually be safer—with support on stairs, ramps, or stepping on and off curbs.

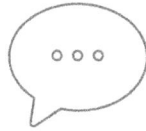

Back in the 1970s, I had a patient who had severe arthritis and pain in her knees. She needed to be using a cane to help her walk more safely and with less pain, but she kept refusing my advice and wouldn't take one home. "It'll make me look old," she insisted. Forget that she was close to 90!

Finally, the day came that her pain became so bad that she surrendered and grudgingly left with a cane.

At her next appointment, she was beaming. Not only was the cane helping her feel more steady on her feet, but someone had tried to steal her purse during a trip to the supermarket—and she sent him scrambling as she beat him with her cane! You can bet she never left the house again without it.

My own mother reacted the same way my former patient had when she started needing a cane, and eventually a walker, to improve her balance. "It will make me look old!" she pouted. My advice to her was, "Carry it with panache, Mom!"—that special sense of elegance and style. "Everyone will wish they had one too," I told her. Well, my mom finally took the coaching and became a proud user of her assistive devices. (I'm sure you've seen people with "decked out" and personalized canes and walkers, making their assistive devices "accessories" and part of their personal style.)

Last, can balance be improved? The answer is yes! People of all ages are able to recover from balance disorders. It is not unusual for individuals—even with a history of balance problems—to regain their control by visiting an appropriate health professional, receiving an accurate diagnosis, and engaging in some form of balance exercises. And while Cate, Dr. Rein, and I can't guarantee you'll never have a fall if you take the advice in this chapter, we do feel confident that you can greatly improve your balance—and your confidence—by using the array of tools we've provided.

Here are some key reminders from Cate to keep top of mind:

* Your **sensory capabilities** (vision, hearing, kinetics) directly correlate with your **body awareness** and, in turn, **your balance.**

* **Sensory information** comes from proprioceptors found in **joints and connective tissue** all throughout the body, sensing where you are in space.

* Exercising muscles and joints and waking the proprioceptors through **movement** and awareness are among the most practical solutions to **reduce your risk of falls.**

* **Feet and ankles** are the base of your body and one of the **primary sources of your ability to balance,** so focusing on ankle conditioning is the most efficient step to move steadier, stronger, and faster.

* **Movement** and **exercise** are powerful steps to lengthen tight tissues and strengthen weak muscles so you can **improve your range of motion** and move, feel, and live better.

Remember: Action conquers fear. You can improve your balance and physical function at any age, given the right exercise and stimulation. Taking action to improve functional abilities and restore confidence is the path toward preventing the vicious cycle of decline, disability, and despair that increases the risk of a devastating fall.

Kudos to you for being proactive on your journey to aging well, moving freely, and living fully!

Chapter 8

Healthy Feet Are
Happy Feet:
How to Keep Them in
Tip-Top Shape

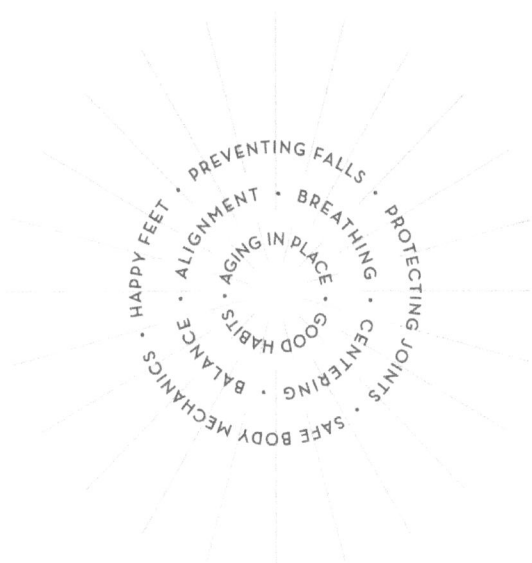

W e talked about giving your feet some love in the last chapter, but in this chapter, I am grateful for the contributions from podiatrist and surgeon Dr. Ross Jenkins. His expertise has allowed me to expand on foot care guidance and address common problems so that you can ensure your feet are happy and healthy throughout your golden years.

We have all heard the term "out of sight, out of mind," and that certainly pertains to our feet. Although they are the foundation for our mobility, balance, and safety, we often don't pay enough attention to them until they begin to hurt. But instead of waiting for aches and pains to draw your attention to your feet, you'll be glad to know there are actually easy ways to give them the care essential to maintaining independence and to preventing—or reducing—pain and injuries.

SIMPLE STEPS TO GOOD FOOT HYGIENE

* Wash your feet daily, preferably with a natural soap that doesn't contain harmful dyes or chemicals.

* Dry thoroughly, especially between the toes, to avoid the growth of fungus.

* Apply a natural lotion, again without harmful chemicals. Take care, though, not to apply lotion between your toes, as it will create moisture that could lead to fungus.

* Further avoid fungus (which likes to grow in moist, dark environments, like shoes) by wearing well-fitted shoes with moisture-absorbing socks. This will help to keep athlete's foot (tinea pedis) and toenail fungus at bay.

* Always trim your toenails straight across and resist the urge to round the corners. Angling the clippers to round the corners may lead to an ingrown toenail.

* Note that as we age, our skin may become drier and thinner, so proper moisturizing and avoiding shoes that rub will help to reduce cracked and painful skin.

MAINTAINING FOOT FLEXIBILITY THROUGH STRETCHING

I don't have to tell you that these days, many of us sit too much. And the more we sit, the tighter our muscles become. We addressed exercises for feet and ankles in the prior chapter to help you maintain flexibility for improved balance, function, and safety—especially when walking—but here we are going to focus on the calf muscles.

The calf muscles are those in the back of your leg that reach from your knee to the back of your heel and are responsible for pointing your foot up and down. Once again, the upward movement of the ankle and foot is called **dorsiflexion**, and the downward movement is called **plantarflexion.**

What occurs when the calf muscles are tight is a more downward-pointed (plantar-flexed) position of the forefoot, with loss of the ability to flex the foot and ankle up into dorsiflexion. This is a special concern for women who have worn high-heeled shoes for much of their lives. When your foot is in a plantar-flexed position, it is difficult to stand and walk with a normal base of support and gait pattern. It causes you to feel like you are falling backwards as your center of gravity moves behind your foot.

Your body's natural response or adaptation to this is to turn your feet out (externally rotate), which unfortunately collapses the arches. This is called *pronation*, and as you might imagine, it can lead to multiple foot and ankle problems—and pain! Some of the issues that can arise are Achilles tendonitis, plantar fasciitis, peroneal tendonitis, posterior tibial tendonitis, sinus tarsitis, and lateral ankle impingement, to name only a handful. Over time, any of these can lead to ankle ligament damage.

Stretching the calf muscle can be done standing (see diagram on page 110). It can also be done when you are seated but may not be as effective.

1. While seated with good spinal alignment, loop a belt or strap under the arch of your foot and try to hold the ends with both hands.

2. Slowly work to extend your knee, while maintaining the pull on your forefoot and that good postural alignment. If you can hold it out in front of you, great! But it is perfectly fine to rest it on an ottoman or stool.

3. Try to hold the stretch for at least several seconds. You should feel the pull in your calf muscle. Be sure you're feeling a stretch, not pain.

(Remember to maintain your good Alignment and conscious Breathing as you do this.)

4. Stretching your feet and ankles on a regular basis will not only help with their flexibility but with your balance too.

COMMON FOOT PROBLEMS AND REMEDIES

Corns and Calluses

Corns and calluses are similar foot conditions, both of which occur in areas receiving friction, usually from your shoes. The problem is that while they both develop as "protective coverings," they can be painful and negatively impact your ability to walk normally.

The difference between the two is that a **callus** is hardened, tough skin you most commonly see over *bony areas* of your feet (typically on your heels, though they can form on any area of your foot, especially the sole). **Corns** are like small calluses, except they tend to form on *soft areas* of the skin, particularly on the tops or sides of your toes. In both situations, the treatment recommendation is the same:

1. Soak your foot for 30–45 minutes in lukewarm water until the skin almost prunes. (The longer you soak the foot, the more moisture the callus absorbs, making it easier to remove.)

2. Use a pumice stone to ease the skin from the callus or corn until it is as smooth as possible, using a light, gentle motion. **Do not rub or grind the stone vigorously.** You want to remove the excess skin gingerly, not create a sore. **Note:** I do not recommend acid or other enzymatic callus removers, which may eat through your

skin. While this is more common in people who are immune-compromised with peripheral vascular disease, it is a much healthier option to use a pumice stone.

For a helpful visual on corns vs. callouses that also includes causes and solutions, the following video is excellent:

https://bit.ly/corns-vs-callouses

A TRICK FOR PAINFUL CALLUSES

Though this may sound like an unusual tip, what follows is an easy way to offload pressure prominences, thus decreasing pain.

- Get a shoe with a removable insole.

- Cover the callus with lipstick.

- Carefully place your foot into the shoe, without smearing the lipstick.

- Stand with your weight on the foot.

- Sit down and remove the shoe.

- Pull out the insole, which now has a lipstick mark that indicates the location of your callus.

- Cut or carve out a hole in the insole around the lipstick mark and voilà! You now have an insole that relieves pressure rather than exacerbates it.

Bunions

Bunions are what are called "bony adaptations in the foot." In the case of bunions, they are bumps that form on the inner side of the foot at the large toe joint. Though they are often hereditary, they are made worse by poorly fitted shoes with a narrow toe box. Luckily, bunions only require treatment—and in extreme cases, surgery—if they are causing chronic pain or are otherwise symptomatic.

Women, in particular, will often sacrifice comfort for style—ouch! But if you suffer from bunion pain, nearly everyone can ease the discomfort simply by wearing shoes that have a more natural foot shape—those with roomier (higher and wider) toe boxes—and avoiding shoes that cramp the toes into unnatural positions.

Hammertoes and Mallet Toes

Like bunions, hammertoes and mallet toes are bony adaptations in the foot. A **hammertoe** is an unusual bend in the middle joint of a toe, while a **mallet toe** affects the joint nearest the toenail, causing the tip of the toe to bend downward at a ninety-degree angle. Both are typically caused by shoes that don't fit well or that force the toes into unnatural positions (as with bunions), affecting the second, third, and fourth toes.

While they may be displeasing aesthetically, the biggest problem with hammertoes and mallet toes is that the bend in the toe joint invites callouses and corns to form. If this occurs, I recommend the soaking and light debridement treatment with a pumice. If painful calluses occur on the tips of the toes, they may benefit from a type of splint, which keeps the toes up and off the ground.

If symptoms persist or you are at high risk for tissue loss, surgical options may be discussed with your podiatrist or orthopedic surgeon.

For an excellent visual that provides illustrations and solutions,
I highly recommend the following brief video:

https://bit.ly/hammer-and-mallet-toes

Ingrown Toenails

We've already discussed the importance of cutting your toenails straight across, not curved, to avoid ingrown toenails, but wearing poorly fitting shoes can be a cause too. In more extreme cases, nail deformities like "pincer nail" may form, where the nail edges curl down, under, and into the skin of the toe, or faulty foot alignment or imbalances may cause the foot to turn in onto the inside of the big toe, causing impingement of its nail into the skin. A foot and ankle specialist may perform a simple procedure to fix either of these problems.

In general, outside of the latter situations, ingrown toenails can easily be avoided by having your nails trimmed by a professional if you are unable to do it safely yourself.

Peripheral Vascular Disease

Peripheral vascular disease (PVD) is a slow and progressive circulation disorder caused by narrowing, blockage, or spasms in arteries that reduce blood flow to leg muscles, often causing pain in the feet. The pain is usually worse at night and may cause cramping in your calves.

If you experience any of the following symptoms, you may have PVD:

* Painful, aching, or tired legs with walking or exercise

* Cramps while lying down (that are often relieved by hanging your legs over the side of the bed or couch)

* Reduced hair growth, or thin/pale skin

* Blue or pale coloration of legs and feet

* Weak pulses, wounds, or ulcers that won't heal

* Blue coloration, severe burning, or thick and opaque toenails

* Numb or heavy feeling in muscles

A circulatory disorder is not something to ignore; however, PVD can often by mitigated or eliminated simply by consuming a healthy diet, doing appropriate exercise, and quitting smoking. In more advanced cases, your doctor may recommend angioplasty and stenting to widen narrowed arteries, or surgery to bypass blocked arteries or repair damaged vessels.

Heel Pain

Heel pain is an inflammatory condition that is most commonly caused by plantar fasciitis, which affects the bottom of the heel, and Achilles tendinitis, which affects the back of the heel. Further causes are bursitis (a condition in which small sacs that cushion the bones, tendons, and muscles near joints become inflamed), peripheral neuropathy, forms of arthritis, stress fractures, and heel spurs, to name a few.

The good news is that heel pain often goes away on its own with home care. For heel pain that isn't severe, try the following:

* **Rest.** If possible, don't do anything that puts stress on your heels, such as running, standing for long periods, or walking on hard surfaces.

* **Ice.** Place an ice pack or bag of frozen peas on your heel for 15 to 20 minutes three times a day.

* **New shoes.** Be sure your shoes fit properly and give plenty of support (revisit the tips in Chapter 7 if needed). If they're worn out or close, it

may be time for a new pair. If you're an athlete, choose shoes that are designed for your sport and replace them as needed.

* **Foot supports.** You can often get relief from heel cups or wedges you can buy without a prescription. (Note that custom-made orthotics are excellent for certain foot issues but aren't usually needed for heel problems.) Do test out foot supports before buying specialized ones, especially if you're planning to spend any length of time with them in your shoes.

If your heel pain lasts more than a few weeks, even after you've tried rest, ice, and other home treatments, and/or you are experiencing one or more of the following symptoms, you will want to see your healthcare provider right away:

* Severe heel pain right after an injury

* Severe pain and swelling near the heel

* Not being able to bend your foot downward, rise on your toes, or walk as usual

* Heel pain with fever, numbness, or tingling in your heel

* Heel pain that persists even when not walking or standing

Athlete's Foot

Athlete's foot is a fungal infection that, as noted earlier, typically grows in areas where there is a moist, damp environment. Symptoms can be itching, cracking, or blistering of the skin, and peeling. While the go-to remedy may be to run out and buy an over-the-counter cream, most of the antifungal products on the market contain harmful chemicals you may not want to use on your skin.

Instead, a little research turned up the following natural remedies, which may not only be more effective but much healthier for you too.

* **Tea Tree Oil**: An essential oil with antifungal properties that makes it a popular natural treatment for athlete's foot. Apply 3 to 5 percent tea tree oil cream or oil to the affected area twice daily. A study published in *The Australasian Journal of Dermatology* found that 10 percent tea tree oil cream was as effective as 1 percent tolnaftate cream in treating athlete's foot.

* **Ajoene from Garlic**: Garlic contains a compound called ajoene, which has antifungal properties. Crush four to five cloves of garlic and rub them over the affected area twice daily. Caution: you may smell like an Italian restaurant!

* **Sosa** (solanum chrysotrichum): This herb has been used in traditional medicine to treat fungal skin infections, including athlete's foot. Apply a cream or ointment made from sosa extract to the affected area.

* **Apple Cider Vinegar (ACV)**: Apple cider vinegar has antifungal properties that can help treat athlete's foot. Simply soak your feet in a foot bath of 70 percent water and 30 percent apple cider vinegar for 30 minutes.

* **Sea Salt**: Sea salt can help reduce fungal growth and inflammation. Mix 1 cup of sea salt with warm water to create a foot bath, and soak your feet for 30 minutes.

Do keep in mind that if your feet or nails have fungus, your shoes have fungus too. You must therefore treat your shoes in addition to treating your skin. If you don't, you can almost count on recurrent fungal infections. You can either use an antifungal shoe spray, or you can put your 70/30 ACV-water mixture into a spray bottle and spray it into your shoes weekly. You may also need to change your socks two times daily if you sweat excessively.

In summary, as you get older, it is a good idea to have your foot health and condition checked by a podiatrist regularly, especially if you have difficulty caring for your feet yourself. You not only want to determine what exercises and self-care you can perform on your own, but in chronic cases, if surgical intervention is recommended or necessary. You don't want to let a long-standing deformity lead to rigid contractures that will be harder to correct. The goal is to keep your feet in tip-top shape for the duration of your life so you can move safely, freely, independently, and as free of pain as possible!

Chapter 9

Boning Up with the Meeks Method: Preventing and Treating Osteoporosis

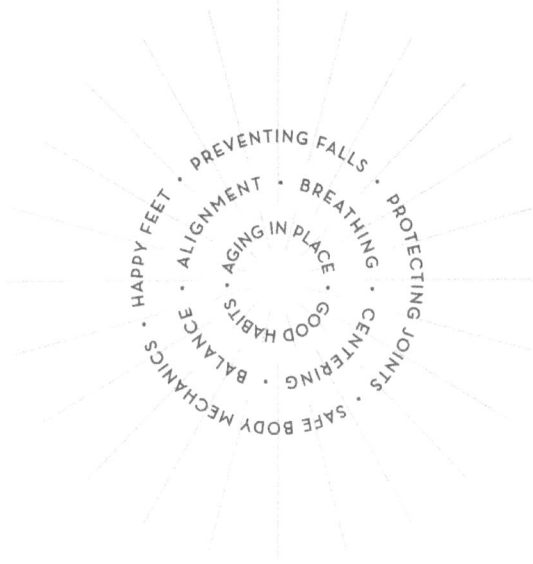

The majority of the following chapter is courtesy of Sara Meeks, PT, MS, GCS, KYT. Sara is not only a highly respected expert in the field of osteoporosis, she is a certified yoga instructor, passionate educator, and physical therapy practitioner. I was fortunate to take several courses with her, and I'm happy to pass on the invaluable knowledge she shares in helping us to prevent—or if necessary, manage—osteoporosis.

The final segment of the chapter was contributed by Clinton Rubin, PhD, SUNY Distinguished Professor of Biomedical Engineering at Stony Brook University in New York. He discusses the benefits of the Marodyne LiV machine, one of My Favorite Things, which was created based on Dr. Rubin's research on the benefits of low-frequency vibration on bone and muscle health.

What Is Osteoporosis?

Simply stated, osteoporosis is thinning of the inner structure of bones.

A host of factors influence a bone's health, the primary ones being nutrition, weight, activity level, medications, and medical conditions. Though we typically hear of the condition in older women, it can happen to men—particularly those who are thin and/or small-boned—and to younger women too. The US Preventive Services Task Force (USPSTF) recommends screening for osteoporosis in women 65 years or older, as well as for younger women whose fracture risk is "equal to or greater than that of a 65-year-old white woman with no additional risk factors."

A diagnosis of *osteopenia*, the early stage of osteoporosis or of osteoporosis itself, is done with a specialized x-ray exam called a DEXA, which must be prescribed by your medical practitioner. Additional tests that indicate the quality of your bones should be discussed with your physician as well.

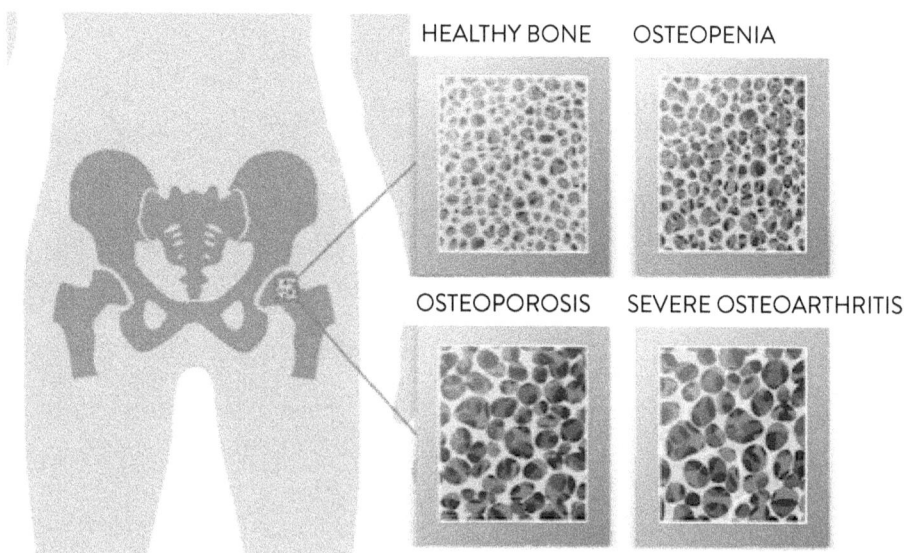

HEALTHY BONE OSTEOPENIA

OSTEOPOROSIS SEVERE OSTEOARTHRITIS

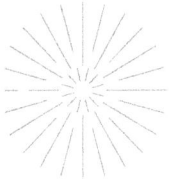

Why Is Understanding Osteoporosis Important?

The strength of your bones is vital. They form the joints that, together with your muscles, produce the movements that get you through your day; your spinal bones (vertebrae) hold the trunk of your body up; and your ribs form the cage that contains your heart and lungs. So when bones become compromised due to osteoporosis, they are prone to fracture. The resulting pain, disfigurement, and/or dysfunction throughout your body that may result can lead to depression, decreased activity levels, decreased socialization, and other life-draining conditions.

This is why your desire to "age safely, wisely, and well" must include caring for your bones—and why this chapter is focused on learning optimum nutrition and exercise techniques to protect them—and you.

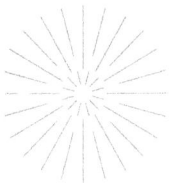

How Do You Manage Osteoporosis?

First, you want to strive for **good nutrition**. Although nutrition is outside a physical therapist's specific professional training, we do suggest you learn the value of integrating whole foods—meaning fruits, vegetables, nuts, seeds, and grains—into your diet. Strive to avoid foods that are processed; most often they contain chemicals that serve no nutritional purpose and are detrimental to your health. Finally, you want to stay well hydrated every day with pure, clean water. (For more on nutrition, see Chapter 11.) Generally speaking, the earlier you start with good nutrition, the better your chances of aging well with fewer health and physical challenges—but it's never too late to get yourself on a more healthful, nourishing path.

Apart from making good nutrition a primary goal, Sara's *Meeks Method* is one of my go-to recommendations. It has been a recipe for success to prevent osteoporosis, and to treat it, at any stage. Preventing fractures is a critical component of her method, and her exercise strategies and techniques are among the most effective you will find anywhere.

The twelve principles to The Meeks Method are illustrated in the diagram below, but we will touch only on Sara's do's and don'ts for exercising with osteoporosis in this chapter.

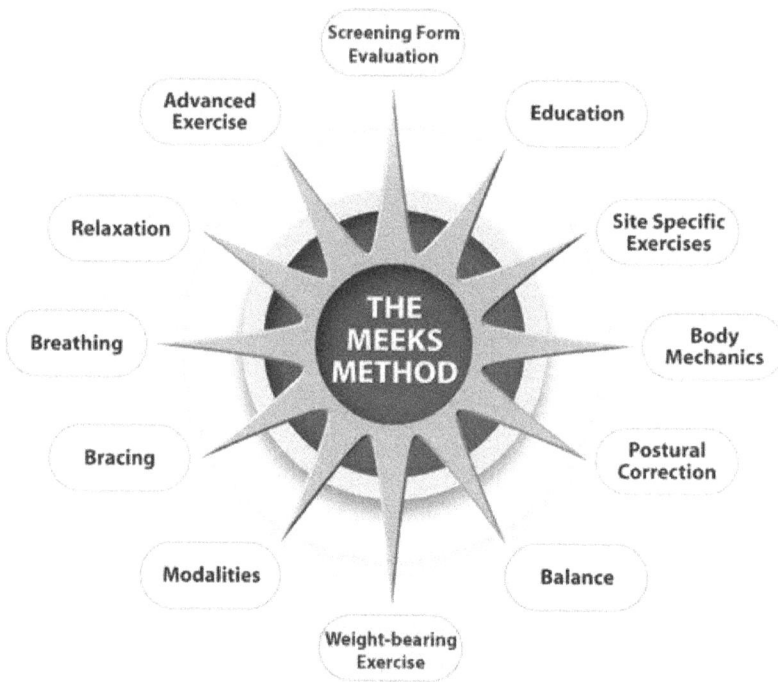

THE MEEKS METHOD

Screening Form Evaluation
Education
Advanced Exercise
Relaxation
Site Specific Exercises
Breathing
Body Mechanics
Bracing
Postural Correction
Modalities
Balance
Weight-bearing Exercise

EXERCISING WITH OSTEOPOROSIS

Preventing the onset of osteoporosis is obviously the goal, but here we will offer valuable tips on the special activity and exercise considerations for the person with osteoporosis, *especially* if you have experienced a spinal fracture.

* As always, begin every exercise with Alignment, Breathing, and Centering, as well as visualizing your intended goal.

* Initiate all exercises lying on your back (supine) to minimize the roll of gravity crushing down on the spine.

* Focus on strengthening the core—the muscles that provide the greatest support to your spine. (Refer back to Chapter 6, the Foot Press Exercise, on pages 82–83.)

* Give focused attention to the muscle groups that correct problem areas, such as a forward head position, rounded shoulders, tight hip joints, etc.

* Stretch tight or restricted joints *after* you have achieved your optimum Alignment.

MAJOR PRECAUTIONS AND NO-NOS

There are three things you *never* want to do if you have osteoporosis:

* "Crunches" or sit-ups—they potentially compress the bones in your upper back (thoracic vertebrae) and can cause the fractures that lead to a hunched back (kyphosis).

* Using machines that supposedly strengthen the abdominal muscles —these also compress the thoracic vertebrae.

* Doing any activity, exercise or otherwise, that increases compression of your vulnerable spinal bones. (Even a sneeze can be an issue if you don't brace your core and keep spinal Alignment.)

SARA'S "DECOMPRESSION EXERCISE"

This particular exercise is beneficial for everyone, and I do it regularly.

1. Lie on your back, with your hips and knees supported at 90-degree angles, with a soft, comfortable support under the nape of your neck to fill in the space, while still allowing for your best Alignment. This position takes away the force of gravity pressing down through your spine and compressing it.

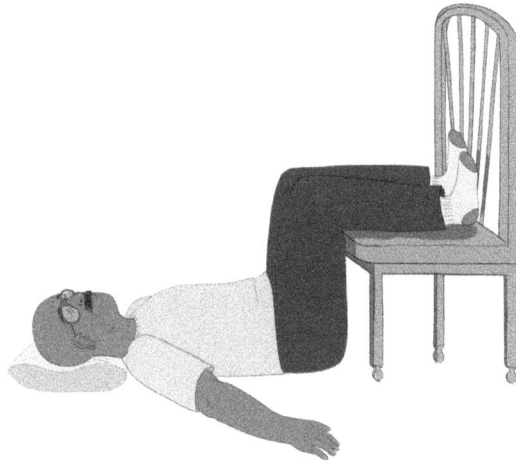

2. Now spend at least 15 to 20 minutes simply doing your *conscious* Breathing and being in a state of relaxation.

Besides taking pressure off your spine and allowing it to realign, this position is excellent for reducing stress and becoming mindful. This is also a perfect time to visualize your body being longer, straighter, and stronger—anything that will make you feel confident about looking, feeling, and functioning well as you age. Sara and I both encourage the use of mindfulness and imagery for helping you manage your mental and physical well-being. This simple activity is a good one for doing so.

Whether you have already been diagnosed with osteoporosis or you are eager to prevent it, I highly recommend visiting Sara's website, which is chock-full of valuable tips and exercises:

https://sarameekspt.com/

BONING UP ON LOW-INTENSITY VIBRATION FOR OSTEOPOROSIS WITH DR. RUBIN

One thing that osteoporosis experts appear to agree on is that exercise is good for your bones. The "use it or lose it" saying is clearly seen in the weakened skeletons of people who can't "use it." Sometimes it's because they have been confined to bedrest, or they've been immobilized due to accidents or illness, where they don't have an opportunity or the ability to apply the weight-bearing and muscular forces that would stimulate bone growth and repair.

On the other side of the equation, athletes enjoy higher-than-average bone quality, with runners, gymnasts, and tennis players having the best. But what is it about exercise—particularly weight-bearing exercise—that is good for your bones?

Researching this issue over the past four decades, Dr. Rubin has determined that the mechanical (physical) forces that occur during exercise provide the needed stimuli for the various types of bone cells.

DID YOU KNOW?

There are several types of bone cells, which form both the hard part of the bone and its softer center—the matrix and marrow. Each cell plays a specific role, including giving the bone its hard structure (osteocytes), cells that create new bone (osteoblasts), cells that re-sorb old cells (osteoclasts), and the mesenchymal stem cells that will ultimately develop into a mature bone cell.

Dr. Rubin's work has gone beyond physical exertion to show that it isn't simply large-magnitude forces, like the ones experienced during vigorous exercise, that drive cell responses. Lower magnitude forces that have less intensity and higher frequency can also have a positive impact on bone growth, and even improve muscular function. This low intensity–high frequency stimulation appears to help limit bone and muscle loss, even as it stimulates musculoskeletal mass.

The devices he helped develop create something like a gentle "buzzing" of bone—or a low-intensity vibration. Over the years, this "buzzing" has been shown to stimulate the osteoblasts (bone-growing cells) and suppress osteo-clast (bone-resorbing cells) in cells grown in the laboratory and in preclinical models. The result of this stimulation was development of bone and muscle cells, even when factors like aging and poor nutrition were working against these goals.

Over the years, Dr. Rubin has collaborated with colleagues around the world to take his research out of the lab and eventually into the clinic. There he has shown that this vibrational substitution for muscle activity (exercise) benefits weight-bearing bones. The clinical trials ranged from boys with Duchenne muscular dystrophy to post-menopausal women with osteoporosis. Treatment involved very low-intensity vibration, which appeared to produce additional benefits of muscle growth and suppressed sarcopenia (loss of muscle mass). Even balance appeared to benefit, plus speeded-up recovery from chemically induced neuropathy in cancer patients. (Other conditions that may eventually benefit from low-intensity vibration are in research trials, as this book is written.)

When asked to summarize his clinical results, Dr. Rubin stated that there is no real substitute for exercise: If you are lying down—sit up! If you are sitting—stand up! And, if you are standing, go for a walk! However, he emphasized that as we age or are confronted with an injury or disease, the musculoskeletal system can benefit from low-intensity vibration. (Of course, proper nutrition is vital as well.)

Finally, Dr. Rubin added that even though his lab focuses on the benefits of vibration for bone structure and function, he warns that high-intensity vibration, such as that delivered by whole-body vibration machines, can be exceedingly dangerous. Those units might deliver up to 10G (10 times Earth's gravitational pull) many times a second. Finding the proper resonance is key.

For more on Dr. Rubin's transformative research on conditions affecting bone and muscle health, and for information on the Marodyne LiV, visit:

https://marodyne.us/

Use code VG200 for a discount.
(Disclaimer: Thera-Fitness collects a commission on
Marodyne LiV when this code is used.)

Chapter 10

Planning to Age in Place? Here's How!

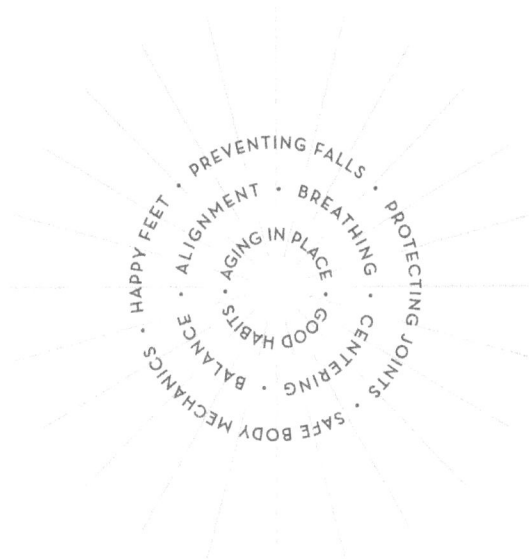

I offer special thanks to Louis Tenenbaum, founder of HomesRenewed.org, and Tara Ballman, executive director of the National Aging in Place Council (NAIPC), for much of this chapter. Along with numerous other professionals and non-professionals alike, their work recognizes that older adults, their children, caregivers, and others have questions about what steps to take to prepare themselves, their homes, and their communities for a safe, independent, and satisfying later stage of life.

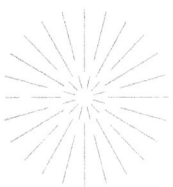

What Is Aging in Place?

There is a common misconception that aging in place means continuing to live in the home you have occupied for years—but this is not true. Rather, it is about the home you *choose* to live in during your later years. That may be a smaller home than the one you have lived in the majority of your life; it may be near the sea, in the mountains, or on a golf course; or it may be a senior community closer to your family. Whatever suits you best, it is about your choice to live where *you* desire—even as your health changes—safely, independently, and comfortably regardless of age, income, or ability level.

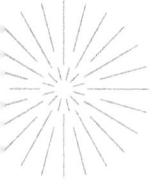

What Is NOT Aging in Place?

Enduring a forced move from the home of your choice because of foreseeable health changes.

Why Is It Important?

Enjoying the bonus of longevity should mean that you're able to make choices that confer dignity, joy, control, respect, contentment, and more. If you are forced to relocate and lose your health at the same time, these high-quality life factors erode quickly. I think we can all agree that added years have no value if we are miserable, broke, or unhappy.

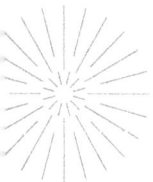

How Do You Achieve It?

The robustness—or decline—of any individual's health is largely controllable by diet and lifestyle. This is why it's so important to eat well, exercise, and to maintain social connections, purpose, and passion. But what happens when we don't do these things, or we never address root causes of symptoms that send us into chronic conditions? Stiffness, slowing down, and further illness and injury can occur, robbing us of quality of life. While no one wants to live in this situation, it's a good idea to prepare the home you have chosen to age in place, in the event you need to accommodate any of these changes—even if temporarily—to not only make your everyday tasks easier on you, but to prevent falls or accidents as well. This is achieved through some simple yet thoughtful planning, as outlined below.

* Include activities such as walking, dancing, gardening, and stretching exercises into your daily or weekly routine (you've learned plenty of good ones in this book!) to improve flexibility and balance.

* Check your home for hazards that can cause slips, trips, or falls and eliminate as many potential trouble spots as possible.

* Don't ignore symptoms that your body is using to communicate to you that something is awry. See a doctor who is focused on determining the root cause, not supplying a prescription to cover the symptom and cause potentially worse side effects.

* If you *are* taking medications, and you're experiencing balance issues, be sure they're not being caused by taking harmful drug combinations.

* Take ergonomics—the relationship between your body and the things you use for everyday activities—into account:

  * Use pots, pans, and other kitchen tools with easy-to-hold handles.

  * Install height-adjustable countertops to help reduce strain on arthritic joints, making meal preparation easier.

  * Purchase lightweight cleaning tools with extended handles to make tasks like sweeping and mopping more manageable.

- For those who love spending time outdoors, ergonomic gardening tools and raised garden beds can help reduce strain on the body while still enjoying hobbies like planting and weeding.

- When it's time to relax, ergonomic furniture and lighting can ensure comfort while reading or crafting.

- Spending time with grandchildren is precious, but as you may already know, it can also be tiring! Having comfortable chairs and sofas with proper back support makes cuddle time more enjoyable, while ergonomic baby gear like strollers with adjustable handles makes outings easier on the body.

In sum, aging in place doesn't have to feel daunting, or even impossible, as you grow older. By incorporating five easy-to-achieve elements—a healthy diet, regular physical activity, social interactions, safety precautions, and ergonomic principles—into your everyday life, you will be well on your way to maintaining your independence and continuing to enjoy the activities you love while aging gracefully in your own home.

For more inspiration and guidance, the following websites offer a wealth of helpful information:

https://ageinplace.org/
https://www.homesrenewed.org/blog/
http://www.louistenenbaum.com/category/blog/

You may also consider obtaining a copy of the book, *Aging in Place Conversations: What Industry Experts Have to Say.* It was published by NAIPC, and I am one of the contributing authors.

Chapter 11

Food for Thought:
Making Nutrition a Priority
for Aging Safely, Wisely,
and Well

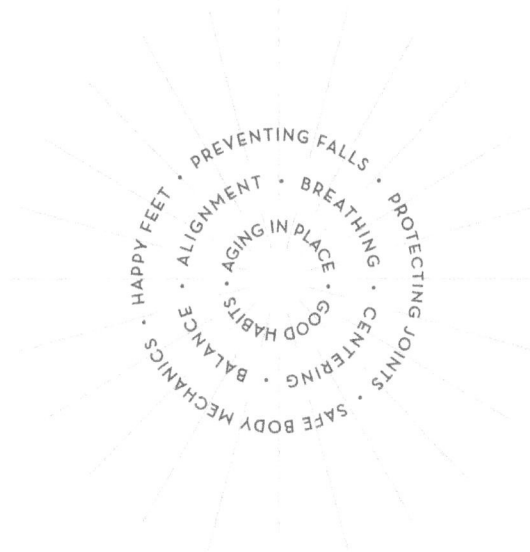

PREVENTING FALLS · PROTECTING JOINTS · CENTERING · GOOD HABITS · AGING IN PLACE · BREATHING · ALIGNMENT · HAPPY FEET · SAFE BODY MECHANICS · BALANCE

I n this final bonus chapter, we address one of the top factors in aging safely, wisely, and well—and that is nutrition.

You've no doubt encountered a plethora of conflicting information over the years about what's good or bad to put into your body. Add to that deceptive advertising, and a proliferation of ultra-processed foods filled with harmful ingredients lining our grocery store shelves, and the confusion only grows. It's no wonder the majority of people are often at a loss for what to eat, and why so many people are unhealthy because of what they are—or *aren't*—giving their bodies in the form of nutrition. While we all know that fast food and many packaged foods fall into the "bad" category, opinions regularly waver on things like salt, sugar, and other common yet controversial ingredients, as well as vitamins and minerals. It can be challenging to consume the right foods if you're overwhelmed and confused!

In this chapter, my good friends Crystal Thackston, CEO of Bridging Wellness, and Stacey Aaronson, a 15-year holistic wellness enthusiast, hope to change that. To cut through the overwhelm, they present the key elements of good nutrition—some of which may surprise you—in an easily digestible (pun intended) way that most anyone can easily apply. Nourishing your body well doesn't have to be complicated, as you're about to find out!

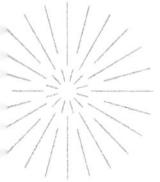

What Is Nutrition?

Nutrition involves a biochemical process that uses food to nourish and provide energy to the cells of your body. It is also responsible for growing and/or repairing structures and organs in your body, like your bones, muscles, heart, lungs, and even your brain. Nutrition is managed through your digestive system, which includes all the organs involved in ingesting, swallowing, chemically processing and absorbing nutrients into your bloodstream, and ultimately eliminating waste.

Why Is It Important?

When you think about your health overall, consider that it is based on two simple things:

1. Having too much of something (chemicals and toxins from air, water, food, pesticides, pharmaceuticals, cleaning products, and personal care products; unhealthy fats and oils; time spent sitting or being immobile; a negative outlook, etc.) and/or

2. Having too little of something (healthy nutrients, pure water, sunshine, healthy fats and oils, vitamins and minerals, exercise, a positive outlook, nurturing relationships, etc.)

The goal, of course, is to strive for the least of the unhealthy elements and the most possible of the healthy elements, so that we're not overloaded—or "underloaded"—with things that create dis-ease within the body.

When we apply this to food, what you take in not only has a major impact on your health, but also on your emotions and well-being. Learning about good nutrition, healthy foods, and solid habits for nourishing and protecting your body are major contributors to your ability to age safely, wisely, and well— and that includes mentally and physically.

Physically, as we age, we start to notice some obvious changes:

*   sagging and crepe-y skin (lack of collagen and water consumption)

*   brittle nails (a slowing in keratin production)

*   muscle weakness (lack of use and lack of nutrients)

*   weakening bones, especially for women (lack of vitamin D and other nutrients needed for bone health)

Though we may not be able to completely stop these natural effects of aging, we *can* slow the process considerably by understanding the basics of good nutrition and by establishing healthy eating habits.

Have you ever experienced uncomfortable situations, like abdominal cramps, heartburn, diarrhea or constipation, or some similar upset of your digestive system? The probability is that the problem was caused by something you ate—or didn't eat, drank—or didn't drink, that your body is either rejecting or in need of. I'm sure you can think of some examples.

Mentally, you can probably think of a time when you were headache-y, sluggish, or "hangry" because you were due for a healthy meal or snack. Did your mental alertness dim? Do you find yourself turning to "drugs" like sugar or a caffeinated beverage to give you energy and mental alertness? (Crystal's confession: I do love my morning coffee, but we shouldn't be reliant on it to get us up and going when we wake up.) And don't forget that your brain depends on healthy carbs from minimally processed, whole foods (more on those shortly) to function properly.

Keep in mind, too, that being awakened from a deep sleep, or being unable to get to sleep, can be from poor choices in what you ate or drank before you went to bed. This is yet another reason that learning about good nutrition is essential for you to maximize your potential—at any age, but especially as you become an "older adult."

Overall, nutritious food gives you mental and physical energy because it feeds the cells in all the organs of your body, enabling them to function optimally—from your brain to your bowels and beyond!

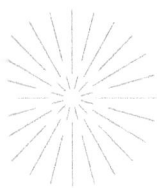

How Do You Achieve It?

What follows are the building blocks of good nutrition—many of which you'll need to "unlearn" from poor guidance and "relearn" here—taken from some of the most cutting-edge natural and holistic doctors and other professionals who are experts in true nutrition.

A good primer is an article in the August 2024 issue of the online publication *Bottom Line Personal* titled "New Science on the Dangers of Processed Foods" (https://bit.ly/dangers-of-processed-foods). It is a real eye-opener about the health risks of additives, as well as excess salt (the bad kind, not the good kind, as you'll read below) and sugar rampant in many American diets.

The sections that follow will help you to make some healthful changes that have the potential to make a big difference in how the cells of your body function—and therefore how *you* function.

WHAT ESSENTIALS DOES THE BODY NEED?

When it comes to what you put into your body, there are really only four essentials for the function of all your cells and organs: macronutrients, micronutrients, proper salt, and clean water. While each person has individual needs—and recommended daily amounts of everything in this chapter will vary and therefore require your own research—by focusing on the basics and getting proper amounts of these four, you'll be well on your way to doing your body a lot of good.

Macronutrients

Macronutrients come in the form of **proteins, good carbohydrates**, and **healthy fats**, some of which have crossover, as you'll see below.

> **Good Sources of Protein** — plant-based sources are healthiest and include: legumes (peas, black beans, kidney beans, lentils, chickpeas), nuts and seeds (pumpkin seeds, walnuts, almonds, chia seeds, sunflower seeds), whole grains (quinoa, brown rice, sorghum), and organic tofu. If you eat meat, consider pastured turkey, chicken, or lean beef, and wild-caught fatty fish, such as salmon, herring, sardines, lake trout, and mackerel.

> **"Good" Carbs** — these are complex and whole, digested slowly, and provide a steady release of glucose (which your body needs for energy) without spiking blood sugar levels. Great sources are:

* whole grains (brown rice, whole wheat bread, quinoa, whole grain pasta)

* fruits (especially citrus, berries, and apples—be sure to eat the skin and seeds of apples too!)

* vegetables (leafy greens, carrots, sweet potatoes, and broccoli)

Healthy Fats — these are naturally occurring fats, not fats from fried or sugar-laden foods. Good fats are essential for nourishing the brain and heart; however, do keep in mind that fats, even healthy ones, **should typically not exceed 10 to 15 percent of your total dietary intake**. Excellent sources are:

* **avocados**

* **nuts and seeds** (particularly pumpkin seeds, sunflower seeds, sesame seeds, hazelnuts, walnuts, and pecans; and nut butters, such as almond and sunflower, in small quantities) Note that peanuts are NOT a nut; they are a legume.

* **fatty fish** like salmon, mackerel, and sardines (Note: Be certain any fish you consume is wild caught, NOT farmed. Even though the oceans are polluted, and there will always be some degree of toxins in wild-caught fish, farmed fish is raised with GMO— genetically modified organism—feed that is highly detrimental to human and animal health. More on avoiding GMOs shortly.)

* **eggs** (including the yolks) Note: Buy eggs from certified humane farms that raise pasture-only chickens whenever possible. Supporting animal welfare is important, and the nutrient value of the eggs is markedly higher as well.

* **flaxseed**

Micronutrients

Micronutrients come in the form of **vitamins** and **minerals,** which healthful, whole foods deliver! However, because our soil has been greatly diminished in nutrients from the overuse of pesticides, you may benefit from supplements to help to fill in the gaps. A great way to know what you need is to have a baseline blood test that measures vitamin and mineral levels, with periodic follow-ups; that way, you won't be over- or under-supplementing products for your individual needs. Again, food is our best source for micronutrients, so don't be tempted to gain the bulk of your vitamins and minerals from a bottle—but they can certainly be helpful in providing some of the elements that are depleted in our food source.

What's crucial to know when buying supplements is that **not all vitamin and mineral brands are the same.** It is imperative to choose reputable, clean, food-based brands so that you don't waste your money—or compromise your health while you're trying to do a good thing—by ingesting tainted, denatured, or cheap vitamins, which are almost always synthetic and do more harm than good.

While we are not being prescriptive about what any one person should or shouldn't supplement, many people do test deficient in certain highly important vitamins and minerals. We've listed the six most common, with the best ways to get them, and the issues most often linked to deficiency.

Vitamin D₃ — considered a miracle vitamin but is actually a hormone!

> *Best Way to Get It*: Vitamin D is made on the skin, activated by a daily 30 minutes of healthy sun exposure on bare skin with NO sunscreen (which is actually laden with cancer-causing chemicals), whenever possible. After exposure, wait at least 30 minutes to shower; you don't want to wash away the activation of the D₃. If you don't have access to daily sunshine, supplementation is necessary.

Issues Commonly Linked to Deficiency: There are a whole host of problems people experience from lack of D3, including but not limited to lowered immunity, weight gain, cancers, heart disease, high blood pressure, and osteoporosis.

Magnesium — the master mineral responsible for over 300 metabolic functions

Best Way to Get It: spinach, quinoa, almonds, leafy greens, figs, avocados, bananas, wild-caught fish, peas, acorn and butternut squash, leeks, alfalfa and radish sprouts, lima beans, edamame, non-GMO whole wheat, and small amounts of fair-trade, organic dark chocolate at 70 percent or higher

Issues Commonly Linked to Deficiency: muscle cramps and weakness, nerve issues, abnormal heart rhythm, fatigue or weakness, high blood pressure, headaches and migraines, and loss of appetite

Vitamin B$_{12}$ — an essential vitamin that the body cannot produce

Best Way to Get It: Because the body doesn't make this vitamin naturally, you must get it from food or supplements. Plant-based foods don't contain B$_{12}$ but animal products do. If you're going to get your B$_{12}$ from meat, strive to choose humanely raised, grass-fed (beef), pasture raised (poultry), or organically fed (pork) with no antibiotics or hormones. If you're vegetarian or vegan, a high-quality liquid supplement once daily will typically suffice. Be sure to purchase the proper form for the body, which is *methylcobalamin*.

Issues Commonly Linked to Deficiency: balance issues, nerve damage, fatigue/ weakness, heart palpitations, hair loss, strange bruising, and dizziness

Vitamin B₉ (Folate) — excellent for skin, gums, and intestines

Best Way to Get It: Folate occurs naturally in asparagus, broccoli, beets, spinach, mustard and collard greens, lentils, eggs, and avocados. If you supplement, be sure not to confuse *folic acid* with *folate*. Folate is the naturally occurring form found in foods like leafy vegetables, while folic acid is the synthetic form added to processed foods and supplements. The body converts folate to the active form of vitamin B9, while folic acid needs to be converted in the liver, which can be slow and inefficient for some individuals. Overall, **folic acid is always synthetic and should NOT be consumed.**

Issues Commonly Linked to Deficiency: low red blood cell count, poor circulation, nervous system problems, mental fatigue, depression, confusion, and insomnia

Iodine — essential for healthy thyroid function

Best Way to Get It: We used to have more iodine-enriched foods in the US, but these days, those foods are rare. The best source of food-based iodine is seaweed, as well as white fish, squid, and oysters. If you rarely eat these foods, a high-quality supplement is a good idea. Do keep in mind that however you take in iodine, an excessive amount can be as detrimental to your thyroid as a deficient amount, so you may want to consult with a knowledgeable healthcare provider to determine the right balance for you.

Issues Commonly Linked to Deficiency: hypothyroidism, fatigue, memory or cognitive issues, dry skin, hair loss, lowered heart rate, dizziness, and cold intolerance

Zinc — plays a key role in skin health, immune function, and cell growth

Best Way to Get It: As with vitamin B$_{12}$, zinc is challenging to get from a plant-based diet, but it can be found in oysters, beef, crab, and other animal proteins. Again, you want to be discerning about the sourcing of your meat and fish. For many people, it is a good idea to get the recommended zinc with a high-quality supplement.

Issues Commonly Linked to Deficiency: slow wound healing, low metabolism, impaired insulin function, unhealthy skin

While this is by no means a comprehensive list, we hope it is helpful in highlighting the vitamins and minerals many Americans tend to be deficient in, so that you can be sure you're not one of them!

Salt

Salt is perhaps the least understood ingredient in the human diet. Our goal in this section is to change that with some empowering education you've likely never heard.

Do you know that your body is about 70 percent saline solution? You heard that right! Every bodily function relies on salt; in fact, it is the third most vital element to the body after oxygen and water. This is why almost 100 percent of the time, a person admitted to a hospital receives a saline drip—salt is actually essential for life. **But it's the *type* of salt that matters.**

What appears on food labels as sodium is *sodium chloride*, or what we call "table salt." This iodized salt has been highly processed, demineralized, potentially bleached, and heated to high temperatures. The result is an element the body doesn't even recognize—yet most canned and packaged foods are filled with it.

We urge you to take a survey of your refrigerator and/or pantry to find out how many milligrams of sodium are in foods you typically consume in a day. Likely, your answer will be "too many." Even the average daily sodium total recommended for older adults is only 1,500 milligrams, which is just under three-quarters of a *teaspoon*. In other words, barely a pinch for an entire day!

Besides the fact that this common ingredient is ultra-processed, the anti-caking agents used in its production actually *leach hydration* from the body. This is why when you eat salty processed foods, or add table salt to a meal, you may become excessively thirsty. Your body is reacting to the loss of hydration, signaling you to drink more water.

So, what to do about getting the requisite amount of healthy salt?

There are a variety of healthy salt options available at almost every supermarket, including Himalayan pink salt, Celtic salt, and gray salt. Each has its own unique profile, with varied amounts of minerals and trace elements. But by far the most exciting discovery is Oryx salt, which you can find out more about at www.oryxdesertsalt.com.

You may find it interesting to look up the respective qualities of each of these different salt sources when you make your buying choices.

A couple of easy ways to use healthy salt include:

* Putting a pinch in your drinking water to create electrolytes (this is particularly helpful after sweating, to replace vital trace minerals, but it is excellent for daily use as well)

* Using in cooking, as a pinch in pasta water, or sprinkling over food

Keys about salt to remember:

* Every function in your body relies on healthy salt.

* We are electrical beings, and salt is a conductor—we therefore need healthy salt for clear thinking.

* Salt is the smallest ingredient in any meal and makes the biggest difference—both in taste and in health impact—so choose the best salt and make it count!

* Any element in excess is dangerous to the body—and healthy salt is no different, so don't be tempted to oversalt your food just because you're using a healthy version. The flavor will be more enhanced with proper salt, so a little goes a long way.

Clean, Pure Water

As we mentioned in the prior section, our bodies are made of 70 percent water, so it's no surprise that the role of water is one of THE most vital for the human body to function. Consider that the body can go without food for days or even weeks, but it cannot go without water for more than 72 hours before our organs begin to shut down. This is why replenishing hydration throughout your day with clean, pure water is of utmost importance.

Unfortunately, as is the case with our oceans, our tap—and even well—water is laden with contaminants. Nearly all US water treatment plants use aluminum and chlorine—both of which are highly toxic to human health. Tap water tests conducted in cities across the nation have found excessive amounts of pharmaceuticals, heavy metals, bacteria, inorganic chemicals, contraceptives, pesticides, unregulated organic chemicals, microplastics, and fluoride—which is a controversial "supplement" for healthy teeth. For this reason, unless you have no other option, no one should be drinking water from a tap without using a filtration system. Many such systems are available to fit varying budgets—from countertop to under-sink versions, as well whole-home systems.

While reviewing the multitude of filtration options is beyond the scope of this book, we urge you to ensure you are drinking the cleanest, purest water you can possibly provide for yourself. What follows are our best recommendations based on a great deal of study on the topic of water.

- ∗ **Avoid store-bought bottled water.** It is filled with harmful microplastics that induce a whole host of issues in the body with potential long-term health effects. If bottled water is your only option, be sure to **never store it in a hot car** or other environment, which leaches further plastic from the bottle.

- ∗ If you have water delivery, strive for **alkaline water,** and be sure the bottles are **BPA-free.**

- ∗ Store your daily water in a **glass** or **stainless steel container** that is comfortable to carry with you—and easy to refill.

- ∗ **Always ask restaurants if their water is filtered.** Many restaurants serve highly unclean water, so bring your own clean water with you, when possible.

- ∗ **Strive to drink half your body weight in ounces every day.** This will keep most people sufficiently hydrated (based on your dietary intake), as well as promote healthy digestion and daily bowel movements. (Ex: weight = 130 lbs times half is 65 = 65 oz. water). Juicy, fresh fruits and high-water-content vegetables (cucumber, zucchini, celery, lettuce, broccoli, cauliflower, bell peppers, and cabbage) are sources of hydration, as well.

TIPS FOR NOURISHING YOUR BODY WELL

Eat Organic and "Whole Foods"

Remember that everything you put into your mouth either hurts or supports your health. While there is certainly a scale—a fast-food burger and French fries made from GMO potatoes and cooked in GMO oil would top the "harmful" scale, while an organic peanut butter and jelly sandwich on conventional bread wouldn't be the best but would fall lower on the harmful end—eating as many organic, whole foods as possible ensures you are in "support" mode more often than not.

Organic produce and other foods labeled organic are healthiest for you by leaps and bounds. Certified Organic farms must go through a formal, rigorous, and lengthy process. This includes adopting organic farming practices—the use of natural methods for pest control, weed management, and soil fertility, and prohibiting the use of genetically modified organisms (GMOs), synthetic fertilizers, and pesticides. Then they must apply to a USDA-accredited certifying agent, submit substantial fees, undergo inspection for compliance, and renew their accreditation via fees and inspection on an annual basis. We tell you this so that you understand why organic is more expensive than conventional. The avoidance of pesticides and GMOs, and receiving nutrients from food grown in healthy soil, is one of the best things you can do to support your health.

Whole foods are "worth their cost" in the same way. These foods experience minimal to zero processing and have the least added salt, sugar, fat, and additives. "Whole" grains, for example, are generally brown and have their fiber-rich bran and vitamins intact, which is ideal for your overall digestion and health. Fresh organic fruits and vegetables are preferred, but canned and frozen organic options offer good nutritional content as well.

When shopping, keep in mind that mainstream grocery stores are laid out with the most heavily processed foods in the middle of the store, with the produce and other bulk or fresh foods in the outer sections. By keeping the majority of your food shopping away from the center of your supermarket, you'll be on your way to a whole-foods diet and lifestyle.

For a helpful list, the Environmental Working Group (EWG) publishes an annual "Dirty Dozen" and "Clean 15," denoting the 12 produce items you should never buy non-organic, and the 15 that are least effected by pesticide use. While organic is always better, if you can't afford to go 100 percent organic, this list is an excellent guide.

https://www.ewg.org/foodnews/

Prepare Your Own Food

Though ready-made or to-go foods are convenient, it is far more beneficial to do your own food preparation, as it is the only way you can control what goes into your and your family's bodies. And—bonus!—it's often more cost-effective as well.

Don't be afraid to try new, healthy recipes. There are hundreds of amazing cookbooks and online resources for vegan, vegetarian, dairy-free, and gluten-free meals that offer delicious alternatives to traditional recipes or takeout favorites. And if you aren't getting enough nutrients from the foods you normally consume, consider increasing their nutritional value by integrating nutrient-dense foods to a dish, such as a dark leafy green like spinach, or a sweet bright red pepper or carrots. The more vibrant the colors, the healthier—and prettier—it will be!

So make that produce aisle your favorite destination at the supermarket and enjoy trying new things.

If you are challenged in preparing your own healthy meals, consider a prepared food delivery service that uses primarily whole and organic foods.

Chew Your Food Slowly and Well

Did you know that of the many functions your body performs on your behalf, digestion is the most labor intensive? Think about it: when food reaches the stomach, it must be broken down by gastric acid before it's sent into the small intestine. This is why it's so important to ease that process as much as you can. There are three important ways to do this:

1. Chew your food deliberately and completely, until it is a paste.

2. Make it a habit to refrain from drinking any liquids 15 minutes prior, during your meal, and 30 minutes after, as liquids (especially cold ones) dilute the stomach acid so necessary for proper digestion. (Frequent bloating, heartburn, and stomach cramps can often be eliminated simply from removing liquids from mealtimes.) Note: this does not apply if you have a hard time swallowing something or may be choking. In those cases, assist your throat with water—or with the Heimlich Maneuver!

3. Avoid taking antacids or acid blockers: they interfere with your natural digestive juices and therefore hamper digestion.

Did you know that **it takes your brain about 20 minutes before it registers that you've eaten**? So it follows that if you're a fast eater, and you haven't given your brain enough time to know it's had enough food, you will likely go back for second servings—and ultimately overeat.

Besides allowing your stomach to communicate satiety to your brain, slowing down also gives you an opportunity to become more mindful of the tastes, textures, and aroma of the food you're eating. It also gives digestion the ability to function optimally from start to finish.

The more you can help that intricate process run smoothly—by chewing thoroughly, not taking in liquid, and avoiding antacids—the fewer digestive issues you'll have, and the better your body will receive all the nutrients it needs.

Whether you're a fast eater or not, here is a method you can use to either slow down or ensure you're eating mindfully:

* Time yourself eating a typical meal, such as dinner.

* Say you consume the entire meal in 15 minutes.

* Your goal is to now stretch a similar meal to 30 minutes. (I realize you may like to eat quickly so your food doesn't get cold, but stay with us here.) There are several ways you can help yourself do this:

  + During your next dinner, set a timer you can see (a smartphone or egg timer works great), and try to employ *S-l-o-w–M-o-t-i-o-n* by chewing more thoroughly (your stomach will thank you!) and eating only half of your entire meal by the 15-minute mark.

  + If you watch TV while you eat, and you are streaming a half-hour program, strive to make the meal last for the entire show. However you time it, you get the idea. The goal is to slow down.

  + Chew each bite of food 25 times. Yes, count! (And again, your stomach will thank you.)

  • Repeat the same timing exercise with breakfast and lunch and adjust your eating/chewing accordingly to achieve between one and a half and twice the time it takes to finish the meal.

The goal is that with time, you won't need the timer, the chew counts, or the program to prompt you to slow down while you eat—you'll simply develop this new habit and reap the benefits as a reward.

FOODS, BEVERAGES, AND INGREDIENTS TO AVOID

When it comes to what you put into your body, the aim is not to be perfect at all times, but to do the best you can to support your health the majority of the time. Our bodies are equipped to handle the bad stuff to some degree, but there are some foods and ingredients you should strive to avoid if at all possible, due to the carcinogenic (cancer-causing) and highly detrimental qualities they deliver to your cells and organs.

If you're not already doing so, start reading the labels of all food you buy and get savvy on ingredients you don't want to be ingesting. Below is a list of those ingredients, followed by foods to be mindful of.

* **any foods—even produce—that are or that contain GMOs.** Common foods that are genetically modified are:
    * **corn** (raw, canned, and frozen; cornstarch; corn syrup; corn oil)
    * **soy** (tofu, tempeh, soybean oil, soy milk, soy protein)
    * **sugar beets** (sugar from these account for about 90 percent of US sugar production)
    * **certain potatoes**

    These foods/ingredients, in particular, should always be organic. On packaged foods, look for the "Non-GMO Verified" label.

* **unpronounceable ingredients** (these are chemicals that should never enter the human body)

* **anything "hydrolyzed" or "hydrogenated"**

* **high-fructose corn syrup**

* **artificial dyes** (look for ingredients like red 3, red 10, red 18, yellow 5, yellow 6, blue 1, blue 2, and green 3) and **"artificial colors"**

* the terms **"artificial flavors"** and **"natural flavors"** (both are usually code words for undisclosed chemicals) Unless a "natural flavor" is

specific, as in "natural vanilla flavor," it's best to either steer clear or to ask the company what their natural flavors are comprised of. Some natural flavors are harmless plant blends used for freshness.

* **aspartame** (a well-documented neurotoxin that causes brain cells to "overexcite" and die) If you chew gum, it likely contains aspartame.

* **soybean, corn, and cottonseed oils** (these are not only primarily made from GMO plants, but are also highly processed and contain high amounts of omega-6 polyunsaturated fats, which are fine in small amounts but not in large ones)

* **bleached all-purpose flour** (bleach . . . need we say more?)

* **table salt** (you already know why!)

* **transfats** (most fried and battered foods; conventional baked goods and baking ingredients, such as cake mixes, frostings, margarine sticks, pie crusts, and shortening; conventional ice cream; conventional beef products; non-dairy creamers; many packaged cookies and crackers)

* **conventional dairy products** (these are laden with antibiotics, hormones, and chemicals that aren't good for animals, and they are equally harmful to humans) Organic nut milks and cheeses, and coconut-based products are more healthful alternatives.

* **conventionally raised / factory-farmed meat** (same note as dairy above)

* **processed meats** (along with the above reasons, these contain harmful nitrates, nitrites, and other artificial ingredients to increase shelf life)

* **canned foods in cans lined with BPA** (a synthetic estrogen). If you buy canned foods, be sure the label says "BPA-free."

* **conventional margarine** (Miyoko's vegan butter is a delicious and healthy alternative to butter; Earth Balance is a good option as well)

* **soda** (besides loads of sugar—and aspartame used in diet versions—the list of harmful ingredients and negative effects on the body from sodas are enough to make anyone want to quit cold turkey)

* **conventional fruit juices** (most "juices" that come in cartons and boxes are mainly concentrates full of processed sugars and other additives. They're not good for your grandchildren—or for you!)

* **Gatorade and other mainstream "energy" drinks** (same as above)

* **non-organic coffee** (coffee beans are the most pesticide-laden crop on the planet, so if you drink coffee, it's vital that it's organic)

* **alcohol** (this has no benefit to the human body, only detriment. Besides leaching hydration, it is highly toxic to cells and organs, particularly the liver and kidneys, our main detoxification organs)

WHAT ABOUT SUGAR?

We're guessing you've heard that an excess of sugar is not your best friend. But are you aware that ingesting added sugar breaks the body down quicker? Crepe-y skin, anyone? But even worse than what it does on the outside, it puts the body into an inflammatory state, which, if chronic, leads to a whole host of diseases. In short, excess sugar makes it more difficult for our bodies to heal.

There are three main reasons sugar has become such a problem in the American diet:

1. Both adults and children consume an average of **100 pounds** of sugar each year, which breaks down to approximately **26 teaspoons of sugar every day**. This largely comes from added sugars in fruit juices, soda,

and sugar-laden processed foods (think cookies, crackers, cereals, and even bread). These sugars added into foods and drinks during processing are those ending in "ose" (lactose, sucrose, fructose, etc.), corn syrup/high-fructose corn syrup, brown sugar, and chemical sweeteners, to name the most common.

2. You now know that **90 percent of sugar comes from GMO sugar beets.** This only adds to the harmful effects of sugar intake from conventionally produced foods, juices, and soft drinks. (If you're going to add sugar to coffee, tea, baked goods, and the like, make sure you're buying/using organic.)

3. In an effort to reduce your sugar intake by choosing **"sugar-free" options,** you are most likely ingesting **artificial sweeteners,** which are actually chemicals. Aspartame is the most common—and most harmful—substitute, used in over 6,000 products and also marketed as Equal, Sugar Twin, NutraSweet, and AminoSweet. If you're trying to go sugar-free, look for or purchase organic natural sweeteners, such as stevia, raw honey, ripe bananas, applesauce, maple syrup, and monk fruit.

Besides the problems of inflammation and the breakdown of cells, excess sugar can also lead to obesity and weight gain, as sugar is stored as fat in the body. The additional weight increases the possibility of further health issues, such as type II diabetes, some cancers, high blood pressure, joint pain (from inflammation), and cognitive decline.

In 2021, Gerontology and Geriatrics Research published a study led by Ballesteros that found aging adults who consume excess sugar in their diets are more likely to have an increase in falling incidents, many of which are injurious. Reducing or eliminating added sugars truly packs a valuable punch!

When you remove added sugars from your diet—even if it's 80 percent of what you typically eat—heart and overall health improves significantly, and weight becomes more easily managed. And just think how much better it gets when you reduce the percentage even more!

Though we've shared a lot with you in this chapter, we want to remind you that nourishing yourself well—despite the challenges in today's food source—does not have to be complicated. It simply takes some relearning and thoughtful attention to what you're putting into your body. We hope this recap and quick reminder list will help you feel empowered as you begin making the most healthful choices you can for maximum benefits.

* Get plenty of healthy macronutrients—proteins, carbs, and fats.
* Get the requisite micronutrients in vitamins and minerals.
* Limit your intake of unhealthy salt and take in a healthful form of salt daily.
* Drink the cleanest water possible, half your weight in ounces daily.
* Eat whole, organic foods as much as possible, prepared at home.
* Chew and savor your food slowly.
* Avoid or eliminate toxic foods and ingredients from your diet.
* Aim to reduce sugar intake by 80 percent, eating only healthy sugars.
* Give your magnificent body love and gratitude daily!

My Favorite Things

I always encourage people to find their own sources of information and inspiration—libraries, the internet, your health and fitness practitioners, even family and friends may have useful tips. But I also want to share some of the programs and products that have impacted my life and that have provided some of the tools I recommend to you. While you should always check resources on any program or product you choose to follow, I hope you will enjoy learning about—and hopefully use—my favorite things, organized by topic.

General Information about Aging Safely and Well

12 Weeks to a Sharper You, by Sanjay Gupta, MD. Lots of good information here and very reader-friendly.

AARP Publications: *AARP Bulletin* and *AARP – The Magazine*

The American Physical Therapy Association/Geriatrics: https://aptageriatrics.org/

Internet Searches—but be diligent about the sources of information. If anything sounds too good to be true and promises a cure for something, please bypass it.

YouTube—Use this site with caution. You can find some crazy things here, but also many highly informative videos. I've included several of them in this book.

NOOM—I like their approach to education and encouragement for those readers looking for a healthier approach to managing their food quantities and choices. I did this for awhile and really liked their use of education and motivational tools and coaching. (You also now have a better understanding about managing your food and lifestyle choices from the chapters in this book.)

Mind-Body Well-Being and Transformation

Kripalu Center for Yoga and Health (https://kripalu.org/) This is where I had my most extensive experience with yoga, which is known to benefit mind and body fitness and well-being. If you can't get there, research local yoga and meditation centers. There are also innumerable books and online programs to help you learn or improve your ability to become more mindful and de-stress, all of which will help you age safely, wisely, and well.

Transcendental Meditation (https://www.tm.org) This training happens to be where I had my first experience with quieting my busy (monkey-brain) mind. As I said in Chapter 1 of this book, you don't need to meditate to become mindful. However, it is a wonderful tool when striving for mind-body well-being.

Landmark Worldwide (https://www.landmarkworldwide.com/) This is the organization that introduced me to many of the strategies and distinctions that allowed me to be unstoppable in the pursuit of my dreams. For anyone wanting a truly life-changing and transformative experience, I highly recommend The Landmark Forum. You can read more about it on their website.

Alignment

Postural Upness and the Vertical Axis of Gravity by my friend and former associate, Howard W. Makofsky. It's a great read for people who want to learn more about posture, what it is, why it's important, and some ideas about how to achieve it. He does reference my ABCs, but differently from the way I promote them. You'll understand the difference if you get the book.

Spinomed (https://www.mediusa.com) This product is a significant tool if any condition is causing you to lose core conditioning and height.

Breathing

The Breather https://www.pnmedical.com/product/the-breather. This product strengthens the muscles of inspiration and expiration. The website has extensive information about the benefits of using it for medical conditions, as well as for improving overall respiratory and aerobic fitness. They are very responsive when you have questions, including why to buy their products, and not the cheaper ones you may find online. I can tell you from personal experience, they work. My aerobic capacity increased and my voice quality improved—especially for singing around the house!

Full disclosure: You get a discount and I get a small commission if you enter the code GOLD-BREATHER at checkout.

Centering

The 3-4-4-3 Technique, described in Chapter 1, can be used to become mindful and to become centered.

Start—Act—Stop (described in Chapter 2) This strategy was adapted from Landmark Worldwide. Multitasking is risky on many levels. Let your mind and body be focused on one task at a time with this SAS technique.

S-l-o-w-M-o-t-i-o-n

Visualize and practice doing an activity in *S-l-o-w–M-o-t-i-o-n* before doing it. Though I realize it's not always possible, try to do it when you can—and remember to prepare for any activity by Aligning, Breathing, and Centering.

The Basic Moves

I have no particular favorite things here, except for you to practice, practice, practice. Use a mirror, if possible, to see if you are keeping your head, neck, and back aligned and your knees behind your toes as you squat.

Balance and Core Conditioning

Motion Stool by Uplift Desk (https://www.upliftdesk.com/stools/) This is only recommended for someone with good balance and coordination.

Pelvic Floor Strong (https://us-pelvicfloorstrong.com/) This is one of many programs for education and training for strengthening the pelvic floor. All exercise programs can be useful if you stay mindful.

Tai Ji Quan Movement for Better Balance (https://tjqmbb.org/) This is a program that provides outstanding training for improving balance. This training is where I really began to appreciate the role our feet play in balance. I recommend searching out an instructor who has learned this approach.

Feet

MoveMor (https://www.movemor.com/) This is the foot and ankle conditioning device that can promote better balance (as described in Chapter 7).

Amazon If you're an Amazon shopper, they have a large selection of aids in helping us keep our feet better aligned and in great shape, such as toe separators, between-the-toe scrubbers, and Birkenstock or Orange shoe inserts, to name but a few. (Other websites have these too, but I find it easy to search Amazon.) Type the item in the search box on the website and have fun deciding which item(s) you want. (If you do not have a Prime membership, make sure you meet the requirements for free shipping.)

Food for Thought

Killer Bees Honey (https://www.killerbeeshoney.com/) I'm highly impressed with the mission of this company and the honey they produce.

General Fitness Programs

Essentrics (https://essentrics.com/) This site has books, videos, and excellent opportunities to "age backwards" using *S-l-o-w–M-o-t-i-o-n* and large-range moves, which lengthen and strengthen the body.

Yoga Body (https://www.yogabody.com/) This site provides excellent total body conditioning in small doses and excellent educational opportunities, where you even have a chance to get your fitness questions answered.

POP-DOC (https://www.pop-doc.com/) This site provides a wide range of well-demonstrated and well-organized exercises. You will notice the model's posture, use of *S-l-o-w–M-o-t-i-o-n*, and correct technique.

General Fitness Equipment

Xiser (https://xiser.com/) This is one of the best products I have ever used for personal fitness, and for achieving outstanding conditioning results for former patients. This hydraulic stepper is portable, durable, and highly versatile. Although it's advertised as a "stepper," it can be used for upper extremity and core conditioning.

Resistance Bands Thera-Band is just one of the many sources of stretch-resistance bands. These are portable with multiple styles and resistance levels, excellent for both stretching and strengthening activities, no matter your level of fitness. Find them online or in your local big-box store, sports shop, etc.

Treadmill My husband and I have a Landice, to which we had full-length handrails attached. I like the additional security when I'm walking or running on it. Research brands that you may like—and that you will use!

Osteoporosis

Marodyne LiV (Low intensity vibration) As mentioned in Chapter 9, this was adapted from a submission by Clint Rubins, whose research led to the creation of this effective device. Though it has not received FDA approval at the time of this writing, I am happy to share that I've had improvements in my own bone density as a result of regular use of this device. Be sure to use discount code VG200 if you decide to order. https://marodyne.us/

Osteo Active Hip Protector This item is sold by CopaHealth. Hopefully, you will never have the fall and hip fracture this is meant to protect you from. Be sure to use the discount code: VGOL1-5. https://copahealth.us/products/osteo-active-hip-protector

Spinomed Though this is not a product I've used, it is one of the products recommended by experts in the field of osteoporosis. It is designed for people who have experienced the unfortunate occurrence of a vertebral fracture, or are at risk of one. Hopefully, you will have learned The ABC Mind-Body System, read Chapter 9 on Boning Up with the Meeks Method, and practiced core-conditioning exercises to keep osteoporosis at bay.

Aging in Place

National Aging in Place Council (NAIPC): https://ageinplace.org

Glossary

This glossary includes the main terms discussed in this book, along with a few that weren't specifically mentioned. In addition, in some cases, I've included comments beyond definitions that I hope you find helpful.

$\ast$

aerobics or "aerobic exercise" — requires oxygen to feed muscular action. Doing activities that cause you to focus on your breathing for progressively longer periods of time, without causing pain or stress, can lead to increased aerobic endurance. Though we didn't focus on aerobic exercise in this book, note that it should be done with medical guidance if you are just starting out. And with *any* exercise program, remember to prepare with The ABC Mind-Body System.

aging in place — thanks to organizations like National Aging in Place Council (NAIPC), older adults and the people who serve them are proactively taking steps that educate and empower individuals' ability to live out their lives in the home of their own choosing.

Alexander Technique — a technique based on the work of Frederick Matthias Alexander (1869–1955), a professional orator who would lose his voice during presentations. Self-study led to the creation of his technique, which increases self-awareness of areas of non-functional muscular tension. As is common in many people, he would unconsciously tighten the muscles in his neck and throat as he spoke, which caused him to lose his voice. This awareness and the eventual ability to release this tension is at the center of his method. Today, Alexander Technique practitioners help clients achieve awareness and release of tension with gentle handling and education. The "open" portion in the Alignment suggestion,—"Lengthen-Open"—comes from my experience with the Alexander Technique.

alignment — refers to the relative position of parts of an object. Good alignment generally allows for more stability in the object and improved function of its parts. That is particularly apparent when it comes to how well our body functions. Think back to the stories and activities in the Alignment chapter.

assistive devices — helpful equipment that can make all the difference in your ability to age "safely, wisely, and well." With a referral from your primary healthcare provider, you can be assessed by a physical and/or occupational therapist. Together they can help you acquire devices or equipment that can facilitate your safety and independence. They can also help you find consultants who can recommend and make adaptations to your home that will promote your ability to "age in place."

autonomic nervous system (ANS) — a type of control center that triggers the release of hormones that either excite or relax the body, engaging the "fight or flight" response mentioned in the book. (Remember, you can exert control over the more negative aspects of the ANS with conscious Breathing.)

balance — refers to an individual's ability to keep Center of Gravity (COG) over base of support (BOS). Standing or walking with a larger BOS improves your ability to balance.

ball and socket joints — allow for movement in multiple planes, such as the shoulder and hip joints.

base of support (BOS) — the area at the bottom of an object. The base of an ice cream cone, for example, is very small, making it impossible to balance, while upside down, the cone is stable because it has a larger BOS. You can improve your ability to balance by widening your BOS.

(The) Basic Moves — a routine of four squatting-related activities that contribute to your ability to bend, lift, and carry objects with lowered risk of accidents and injuries.

body mechanics — relate to the way your body moves when you are doing physical tasks. Good body mechanics include maintaining your Alignment, Breathing, and Centering and following the principles outlined in Chapter 2. Using good body mechanics contributes to less pain and joint damage during bending, lifting, and carrying activities.

Breathing — a function of the respiratory system (see "respiration" below). Correct breathing patterns optimize the intake of oxygen and the output of carbon dioxide. Breathing occurs automatically; however, you can *consciously* control it, which is a significant factor in mind-body well-being.

carbon dioxide — the gas produced after oxygen has been taken out of the blood and used for cell metabolism.

Centering — a concept that refers to the mind and body working together, as opposed to your mind doing one thing while your body is doing something unrelated to what you're thinking about.

center of gravity (COG) — the point in your body around which balance occurs. When you are standing, it is generally just behind and below your belly button, or navel.

concentric contraction — one in which a muscle shortens as it works to overcome resistance.

condyloid joints — those that allow for gliding and circular movement, such as the wrist and ankle joints.

conscious breathing — refers to paying attention and taking control of your breathing.

COPD (chronic obstructive pulmonary disease) — a condition in which there has been damage to the lungs. People with COPD tend to struggle to get adequate oxygen into their bodies for cell metabolism, and also tend to not fully exhale carbon dioxide. Endurance for activities becomes a big issue for these individuals, but breathing exercises can help.

core conditioning — the strengthening of the muscles that encase the torso, top, bottom, front, and back. These include the deeper abdominal and back muscles, diaphragm, and pelvic floor. Conditioning the core tends to improve posture and help minimize back pain, among other benefits.

corns and calluses — among several issues affecting the feet. If not carefully managed, they can cause pain throughout your body and impact your ability to walk and balance well.

DEXA (dual energy X-ray absorptiometry) — one of several tests that can analyze the integrity of your bones, meaning how dense and healthy they are. Men and women should discuss getting tested with their healthcare practitioners. If osteopenia or osteoporosis is detected, there are many actions to take to prevent the risk of falls, fractures, and other potential complications from the condition.

diabetes — a disease related to your body's ability to metabolize sugar that can be easily managed and/or reversed with proper nutrition. If not managed, it can affect many systems of your body and impact your ability to "age safely, wisely, and well."

diaphragm — the primary muscle of respiration (breathing). Shaped like a dome curved up into your chest, when it contracts, it flattens, creating a negative pressure in your chest cavity, which then sucks air into your lungs. The flattened diaphragm presses down on the organs below, causing them to protrude.

diaphragmatic breathing — efficient use of the diaphragm, as opposed to other muscles that also relate to breathing, such as muscles in the neck, shoulders, and rib cage. Diaphragmatic breathing is sometimes referred to as "belly breathing" because the abdomen will protrude with inhalations as the diaphragm contracts and flattens.

dynamic balance — what you are doing as you are moving and keeping your balance. Your Center of Gravity (COG) continuously travels over your Base of Support (BOS) as you move.

eccentric contraction — the lengthening of a muscle as it controls a movement. Lowering a bent elbow occurs as the bicep muscle lengthens, versus what happens as it contracts to bend the elbow.

endurance — the ability to do an activity over an extended period of time. It is impacted by the health of multiple systems in the body, especially the heart and respiratory systems. In most cases, you can increase your endurance by increasing the number of times or length of time you do an activity.

equilibrium — being in a state of balance and often used interchangeably with the word balance.

ergonomics — the study of the interaction between you and your environment. Ergonomists are able to help people and companies provide for the physical and mental safety and well-being of individuals.

exercise — often a hated practice, unless you find the activity fun! It is usually prescribed by the number of times an activity is done (repetitions/reps) and how many times those reps are repeated (sets). For example, raise a weight, or sit and stand from a chair, in three sets of ten repetitions. You can turn any of your everyday activities into "exercise" by doing them in X number of sets, each set having X number of repetitions. Documenting your number of sets and repetitions lets you track your progress. Additionally, exercise may encompass a physical activity performed for a period of time, such as dancing, hiking, yoga, Pilates, etc.

exhalation — the process of removing stale air from the lungs. It can be done through the nose or mouth, but most important is to do it *consciously* when using it to calm the body and mind, and to do prolonged exhalations with pursed lips, as outlined in Chapter 2.

fear of falling — a common mindset if you have balance issues. Strategies for managing this fear include being assessed for an appropriate assistive device and using the self-talk strategy, "I am tall, strong, and confident."

Feldenkrais Technique — an approach to mind-body fitness and well-being based on the work of Moshé Feldenkrais (1904–1984). As with related approaches, it promotes conscious performance of movement and release of habitual patterns of tension, which allows for greater freedom, comfort, and efficiency of movement.

fight or flight — your body's reaction to fear, whether real or imagined. The danger to your well-being occurs when this reaction is habitual, or chronic. Performing conscious breathing, reciting the Serenity Prayer, and distinguishing whether a situation is "life or death" can be highly effective for helping you manage this reaction.

flexibility — can refer to your mental as well as physical condition. Can all your body parts move through their full ranges of motion? Is your mind flexible and open to new ideas? Working on both is part of transformation.

functional fitness — refers to converting your everyday activities into exercise by adding sets and reps. Traditional exercise often involves doing an activity, like lifting a barbell, which can certainly improve your strength, but not guarantee that you will improve your ability to get out of bed.

gait — the way you walk, analyzed according to the length of your steps (stride-length), the width of your base of support (BOS), your ability to walk with a heel-to-toe pattern, the speed with which you walk, and other things related to "normal" walking.

glide joints — allow for gliding movement, such as the joints between the bones of the spine.

hinge joints — allow for bending and straightening movements, like at the distal finger joints. The elbow and knee joints are mistakenly called "hinge joints," but they have gliding movements as well. Pure hinge joints are rare.

imagery — an excellent tool to train your mind and body for better performance of an activity. It is related to visualization, where the things you imagine can directly affect how your body responds. It is equally beneficial for managing, and even creating, greater well-being.

inhalation — the process of taking air in. It is always best to inhale through your nose, where air can be filtered and warmed or moistened. I recommend you research the many benefits of breathing in through your nose.

intentionality — though we don't touch on this in the book, it is what you aim to accomplish when you take on a project or an activity (such as reading this book!).

isometric contraction – where a muscle tenses without getting longer or shorter. Think of holding something in one place, neither lifting or lowering it, or squeezing a specific muscle. That is an "isometric." When a lot of force is used during this type of contraction—straining to lift a weight, or even on the toilet—it is critical to maintain a breathing pattern to avoid increasing your blood pressure, which could have life-threatening consequences.

joints — the link between two bones that allow for movement. Managing your Alignment as you move is one of the keys to keeping your joints pain-free and functional throughout your life.

joy — a feeling you experience when there is love, health, and purpose in your life (this author's definition!).

kinesiology — the study of human movement, which includes physiological, anatomical, biomechanical, pathological, and neuropsychological principles. Much of The ABC Mind-Body System comes from the study of kinesiology.

kinesthesia — your body's ability to sense where it is in space (here on Earth). There are nerves specifically designed to detect how and where your body is moving. They then make necessary adjustments so you can keep your balance, accomplish a task, and keep from falling.

Landmark Worldwide — comprises a series of seminars that promote the development of personal growth and transformation. Many strategies presented in this book are derived from these seminars.

longevity — refers to the length of your life. I hope this book will help you achieve a long, healthy, and productive one!

meditation — a formal system for achieving mindfulness. There are many systems of meditation with various intentions; however, you can be mindful without meditating, which is one of the skills I hope you took from this book!

(The) Meeks Method — a 12-step approach for prevention and/or management of osteoporosis created by Sara Meeks, PT. (Be sure to check out her many YouTube videos.)

metabolism — the complex series of chemical reactions in your body that enables your cells to extract the nutrients they need to function—and thrive!

mind-body — refers to the way the mind influences how the body functions, while the condition of your body impacts the way your mind functions, including your thoughts, feelings, attitudes, etc. An example is being "hangry"— the word people use if they get angry when they are hungry.

mindfulness — the state of awareness you have when you are fully conscious of how and what you are feeling and doing. You are less likely to have an accident or make a mistake if you are being mindful.

mnemonics — those sometimes cute, but effective tools to help you remember things. Thera-Fitness uses an ABC mnemonic to help you learn the basics of safe, efficient mind-body fitness and well-being.

neuroplasticity — the miraculous feature of human beings that allows us to grow and learn until our dying days. That's why you can teach an old dog new tricks!

nitrous oxide (NO) — a gas produced in your nasal cavity when you inhale through your nose. Your body benefits from NO because it increases blood flow through your lungs and boosts oxygen levels in the blood. That increased oxygen level can improve your energy level and endurance.

occupational therapy — a medical profession that often works in partnership with physical therapy to optimize a person's ability to achieve functional safety and independence.

osteoporosis — a condition of weakened bone structure with many potential causes, not limited to older women. Managing your posture and nutrition are only two factors related to preventing or managing osteoporosis. Sara Meeks's work covers many more.

oxygen (O$_2$) — the gas required to fuel all cellular functions (metabolism) in the body. You may hear it referred to as "cellular respiration." Diaphragmatic breathing through the nose is recommended for optimum oxygenation of the blood.

Parkinson's disease — a condition that causes abnormal function of the neuromuscular system. It affects a person's ability to control their movements and puts them at a greater risk for falling.

pelvic floor — the lowest part of your trunk that contains all the muscles that allow us to control our urinary, bowel, and some aspects of our sexual function. It also forms the bottom portion of our "core" and benefits from being exercised, just like the rest of the core muscles.

personal growth — what occurs when you expose your mind and body to new or challenging ways of thinking or behaving. It requires a willingness to let go of preconceived ideas of right and wrong, and good and bad, although you may wind up with firmer convictions in your beliefs.

physical fitness — relates to you having the flexibility, strength, balance, and endurance beyond what you need to perform your everyday tasks. It is generally accomplished with exercise, including "functional fitness."

physical therapy — the profession specialized in analyzing human movement and function. Physical therapists and physical therapist assistants have the necessary education and training to assess and ultimately treat conditions that may create dysfunction and disability in an individual.

Pilates — an approach to mind-body fitness with a primary focus on core conditioning, control, and breathing. It was developed by Joseph Pilates, a German physical trainer, who was aware of the relationship between mind, body, health, and well-being.

pivot joints — such as the one between the top two vertebrae in the neck that allow your head to turn around a single axis. See how it works at https://bit.ly/pivot-joint-demo

power — an element of physical fitness that is not a typical part of a fitness routine. It involves heavier weights and fast repetitions that tire out the muscles. Most of us are not going to do that type of exercise, unless we are a competitor. (Senior Olympics, anybody?)

progressive resistance — the building up of weight that has to be over-come to achieve an exercise or task. You may initially be able to lift an item of one pound. With progressive resistance exercises, you track how much weight you are increasingly able to lift or move. Progressive resistance can be achieved by how many times you can lift your own body weight—or by using more challenging weights or resistance bands. (See "Repetitions" and "Sets.")

proprioception — your body's ability to sense where it is, what it is doing, light and touch pressure, etc. It combines with other systems in your body and plays a large role in your ability to maintain your balance.

pulmonary hygiene — involves a series of actions, like deep breathing, coughing, and positioning your body in ways that allow you to clear your lungs of stale (residual) air and secretions, which take away space your lungs need for oxygen. (Diaphragmatic breathing helps the process of pulmonary hygiene.) This is especially important if you have a lung condition like COPD.

purpose — the sense of mission, or something you are committed to accomplishing, that often gives your life meaning and a reason to do everything you can to age safely, wisely, and well!

pursed lips — pressing your lips together as you exhale creates backward pressure to the air coming out of your lungs. This helps to keep air passageways open and is a useful technique if you have a condition like COPD, where air passages may tend to close during exhalation.

range of motion (ROM) — a measure of flexibility, describing how far and in what directions a normal joint can move. Stretching is the technique used to improve joints with limited ROM.

reactions and reflexes — automatic movements your body makes in response to some stimulus. Movements to maintain equilibrium and "fight or flight" are reactions, while a blink and a knee jerk are examples of reflexes. Though you may be able to limit your body's reaction to something, reflexes are generally not controllable.

repetitions — the number of times you do an activity or exercise. Your ability to improve your physical fitness often depends on progressively increasing your number of repetitions and/or number of sets, in addition to increasing the amount of resistance against which you are working.

residual air — the air that sits in the corners of your lungs, like dust bunnies in the corners of closets. Diaphragmatic breathing with prolonged, pursed-lip breathing is a strategy for clearing your lungs of those dust bunnies, leaving more room for oxygenated air.

resistance — a force that has to be overcome. When you are working to increase your physical or functional fitness, you need to make your muscles work against resistance. That resistance can be your own body weight, or an outside resistance like a barbell, a can of beans, or resistance bands—anything you have to work to lift or move.

respiration oxygen for cellular respiration — extracts energy by the reaction of oxygen with molecules derived from food, and produces carbon dioxide as a waste product.

respiratory system — includes everything from your nose, past your throat (pharynx), into large tubes called bronchi, down to smaller tubes called bronchioles, and finally into the air sacs of the lungs themselves. The diaphragm is the muscle that helps bring air into the lungs. When the diaphragm relaxes the air is expelled, often with a little help from the abdominal and rib cage muscles.

saddle joints — allow for a unique gliding and rotating movement, such as that found at the base of the thumb. Here's a brief look: https://bit.ly/saddle-joint-demo

self-talk — the things you say to yourself, consciously or unconsciously, silently or out loud, that have positive or negative effects on how your body feels and functions. Once you are aware of them, you then can make a choice to change them to something positive. ("I am tall, strong, and confident!") Many of us not only mistake our negative self-talk to be real or true, but we use the "forbidden words" of "should," "shouldn't," "can't." By transforming your self-talk, you can transform what's possible in your life!

sensory systems — the way your body gets the information it then uses to make decisions; make (automatic) adjustments to what you are doing and how you are doing it; have reflexes or reactions, and more. There are five common senses: vision, hearing, smell, touch, and taste, along with the sixth sense of intuition, also called extra sensory perception.

(The) Serenity Prayer — a non-denominational prayer, not connected to any religion, that has existed in some form since ancient times. Today it is basic to all 12-Step programs, such as Alcoholics Anonymous. It is useful in circumstances where you are struggling to make a decision about something, and it can be very helpful in making a distinction about how and whether you should take any action. It reads: "G-d grant me the serenity to accept the things I cannot change; the courage to change the things I can; and the wisdom to know the difference."

sets — the number of times you perform a group of activities ("repetitions"). In progressive resistance exercises, you can add sets, repetitions, and resistance to force your body to work harder and get stronger.

S-l-o-w-M-o-t-i-o-n — the part of The ABC Mind-Body System that is encouraged to help you learn a new skill, to improve your strength and balance when doing a physical/functional activity, or to help you de-stress and maybe even prevent a fall or injury. One trick for slowing down is to say the words *S-l-o-w–M-o-t-i-o-n* as slowly as you can. It will make you laugh, but it works!

SMART goals — Specific; Measurable; Attainable; Relevant; and Time-based.

spine — made up of 24 bones (vertebrae), giving it shape and structure. Discs between each vertebra function like shock absorbers, while "facet joints" allow for the spine's flexibility. Ligaments hold the spinal structure together, and muscles provide the force for spinal movement. Learning how to protect these structures using the Basic Moves can help you prevent pain and injuries.

squats — the movement of bending and lifting, like when you sit in a chair, or bend to pick something up from the floor. Correct technique can help prevent pain and injury, as good postural alignment is maintained and strong thigh and buttock muscles do the heavy lifting. (Review The Basic Moves.)

stability — occurs when there is no movement and the Center of Gravity (COG) stays over a person's or an object's Base of Support (BOS).

strength — the quality of your muscles that enables you to do the bending, lifting, and moving that make up your everyday life. Strength increases as you do activities that cause you to overcome resistance, such as the force of gravity as you sit and stand, or barbells, resistance bands, etc. Managing the amount of resistance, as well as the number of repetitions and sets, all contribute to strength-building.

stress — a response to a potentially negative event, real or imagined, that causes a mental and physical reaction in the body. Common feelings associated with stress are worry, anxiety, fear, upset, anger, etc., all of which are highly detrimental to the body when the response is chronic. Conscious breathing is an excellent remedy, as is positive self-talk.

stretching — a technique to increase your joint flexibility (range of motion). Yoga provides a generally safe, effective approach to stretching, because of how it integrates breathing with the method.

tai chi — an ancient Chinese martial art that is a gentle, low-impact form of exercise in which practitioners perform a series of deliberate, flowing motions while focusing on deep, slow breaths. Often referred to as "meditation in motion," tai chi aims to concentrate and balance the body's *qi* (vital energy), providing benefits to mental and physical health.

toes — play a substantial role in your ability to walk pain-free, to balance, and hopefully prevent falls. Toes are not given enough respect by most people, so be sure to give them some love by maintaining their strength, flexibility, and skin condition!

transformation — making a significant change in mind, body, or spirit. This book, for example, aims to educate, inspire, and empower you to make transformational changes that might lead you toward a longer, healthier, and more fulfilling life.

upset — a reaction to the thought that there is something wrong with you, someone else, or a circumstance. Landmark Worldwide provided this description of the three things that are usual sources of upset. See how any one of these may be true the next time you are upset.

1. A thwarted ambition. You wanted or planned to do something, but something got in the way.

2. An unfulfilled expectation. You expected something would happen, and it didn't.

3. An undelivered communication. You want or need to express something to someone, but for some reason you didn't, or haven't. (Thank you, Landmark, for helping us make these distinctions.)

vagus nerve — the main nerve of the parasympathetic nervous system, which controls specific involuntary functions in the body, such as digestion, heart rate, lymph movement, and the immune system. The vagus nerve is critical to understand because it is the longest nerve in the body, with branches that touch nearly every internal organ. It extends from the brain stem all the way to the gut, or lowest part of the abdomen, essentially communicating everything that's happening in the body to the brain. When you are stressed, whether by an actual threat to your life or by any number of daily stressors, your body goes into "fight-or-flight" mode. When this occurs, the parasympathetic system shuts down. In other words, your body puts all its resources into saving your life in the moment of real threat, and in so doing takes resources away from digestion, immunity, etc.

What you may not realize is that when you internalize stressful situations on a regular basis, your body doesn't know the difference between stress from a real life-threatening situation (dodging a speeding car, running from a pursuer, etc.) verses stress that is self-imposed due to personal upsets, like work, children, traffic, world events, and the like. When stress is chronic, meaning it is long lasting or perpetual, your involuntary nervous systems are suppressed. It's no wonder, then, that chronically stressed people are often plagued with digestive issues, immune deficiencies, heart problems, and other serious concerns. It's that mind-body connection in action—you are telling your body that you're effectively "running from a pursuer" all the time, nearly 24/7.

But when you breathe consciously, you communicate to your vagus nerve and parasympathetic nervous system that all is well, which automatically instructs all of your systems to function normally. This is why the way you breathe and doing conscious breathing are vital to keeping you healthy and alive.

vertebrae — the little bones that make up your spine and help to hold you erect. Good nutrition, erect posture, and strong body mechanics help to keep them from succumbing to the challenges of osteoporosis, including fractures and postural deformities.

vestibular system — made up of structures in your ear that communicate with your brain. They tell your body how and where your head and body are positioned or moving. Damage to any part of this system can cause you to be dizzy and at risk of losing your balance. Physical therapists, and eye, ear, and nose specialists can evaluate and suggest appropriate treatments for problems with this system.

visualization — your ability to picture something in your mind, similar to imagery. You can create images on your own or have them suggested to you by someone else, in person, on tapes, in videos, etc. They are a great gift to you because they can help you create positive mental and physical states of well-being. (Isn't that what we are all striving for?)

weight-bearing exercise — a method of increasing your physical fitness by using the weight of your body as the only resistance. Doing push-ups, and sitting and standing from your chair (squats), are two examples of weight-bearing exercises that are important aspects of your functional fitness.

weight-shifting — shifting your body's COG over changing bases of support (BOS), as opposed to staying in one, unmoving, stable position. It is a necessary skill for normal balance and the ability to walk with a normal gait.

yoga — considered a mind-body practice because it integrates movement, breathing, and mindfulness. Elements of yoga are found in the stretching methods promoted in this book. Many mental and physical benefits derive from yoga, especially when precautions are taken to avoid stressing osteoporotic bones.

Acknowledgments

There is no book I know of that doesn't come to life without the aid, inspiration, and support of a community of people. In my case, many of those people are part of my past, while others stand beside me today. I can't express enough the depth of my gratitude to not only these individuals, but also to the life experiences that contributed to the knowledge and understanding that continue to enable me to "age safely, wisely, and well"—so far.

I'll begin with my parents, Goldie and Julie Gold. Mom was always there providing support, guidance, and inspiration as I made my way through school. Her typing and editing skills made my essays and eventual Master's thesis look great. Dad provided more of the fun and daring risk-taking skills that have helped me take on challenges beyond what might be expected of "a girl," "a woman," and especially an "older woman." I wish they were here so I could share my joy at completing this book and continuing to fulfill my dreams.

Still in the past are my late brother Lonnie, who, in spite of being profoundly mentally retarded and nonverbal, lit up my life and the lives of anyone who had the good fortune to meet him. Joyce Alexander was a classmate and one of the last victims of polio just as the vaccine for it came out. Even with her profound physical challenges, Joyce became an artist and the second person who helped me develop a sensitivity to people with disabilities. I also acknowledge Camp Carola, which served children with physical challenges. In the summer of 1963, while I was a camper at Surprise Lake Camp in New York, we had a visit from Camp Carola. One of their counselors noticed how at ease I was with the children in wheelchairs, assistive devices, etc., and suggested I consider becoming a physical therapist. The rest is history.

The following people from my professional background stoked my passion and transformed my practice of physical therapy. Those early former professors, department heads, and all-around inspirations included: Elizabeth

C. Addoms, Dr. Arthur J. Nelson, Dr. Robert Bartlett, Mr. Ted Corbitt, Dr. Marilyn Moffat, Dr. Robert Ayres, Dr. Stanley Paris, Ms. Margaret Knott (PNF), Ms. Dorothy Voss (PNF), Mrs. Berta Bobath (NDT), and too many more to mention. Additionally, Dr. Renato da Costa Bonfim arranged for me to live and teach in Sao Paulo, Brazil, at the Associação A Crianças Defeituosas (AACD). *Tengo saudades* (I miss you).

More recently, I acknowledge those who have made this book something we can be proud of and that will make a difference in the lives of its readers. First, there are the professionals who contributed to its content: Dr. Rein Tidieksaar, Ms. Cate Reade, Dr. David Neuman, Dr. Ross Jenkins, Dr. Matt Jeffs, Ms. Sara Meeks, Dr. Clint Rubin, Ms. Tara Ballman, Mr. Louis Tanenbaum (NAIPC), and my friend Crystal Thackston.

On the book production end, there is not enough gratitude for its publisher and my friend, Ms. Stacey Aaronson (www.thebookdoctorisin.com), and our illustrator, Ms. Lily Padula (www.lilypadula.com), whose work I had admired for many years, never dreaming I would be blessed enough to work with her. Stacey has stood by my dream of writing a book for more than ten years and never failed to assure me it would come to fruition one day—and here it is! Thank you also to Carmen and Jon Eckard (https://eckardphotography.com/)/', whose photography has made me look my best as I enter my eightieth year. I am grateful. And finally, no one would even know about me and this book if it weren't for my marketing guru, Melanie Diehl (www.melaniediehl.com) and audio guru Vaughn Fahie (www.thevoicebrander.com).

Of course there are family, friends, and neighbors who have been cheering this project on—but no one like my husband, Tom Carbone. He has been the "wind beneath my wings," as they say. His love, devotion, and commitment to me, this project, and our lives is unsurmountable as we both strive to age "safely, wisely, and well." Thank you, my love—forever and ever.

Finally, I would like to thank and acknowledge you, my reader, for taking on the mission of living your best life physically and mentally. I hope you will take time to let me know how you are doing.

About the Author

C. Vicki Gold, PT, MA, considers herself lucky to have been born in Phoenix, Arizona, where she learned to love the great outdoors. The birth of her profoundly developmentally delayed brother, Lonnie, brought Vicki's family back to their roots in New York, and the later loss of a dear childhood friend to polio primed her for an eventual career as a physical therapist. Her passion and dedication to her chosen field led her to specialize in neurophysiologic approaches to therapeutic exercise (PNF and NDT, specifically) as well as in geriatric rehabilitation and fitness.

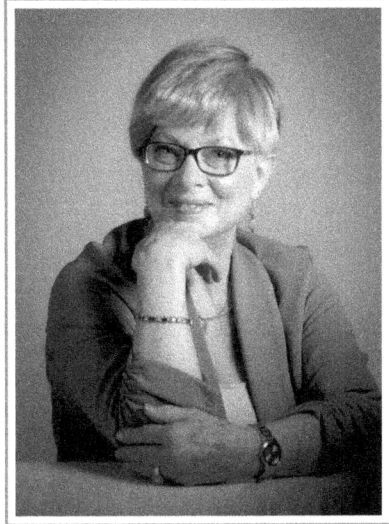

Vicki's background included her perpetual quest for challenging and enriching experiences, among them: director of the Physical Therapist Assistant Program at LaGuardia Community College in NYC; director of the physical therapy department at AACD in Sao Paulo, Brazil; marketing manager at Invacare; and faculty positions in several physical therapy programs in New York and California.

In addition to her traditional medical background, Vicki has had extensive experiences related to mind-body fitness and well-being: yoga, Pilates, tai chi, Alexander and Feldenkrais Techniques, Landmark Worldwide, and work with cognitive behavioral therapists among them. Combined with her eighty years of life experience, Vicki hopes the material in this book will give the reader the inspiration, education, and empowerment to live their lives "safely, wisely, and well."

Reach out to Vicki with questions or comments at
vicki@thera-fitness.com

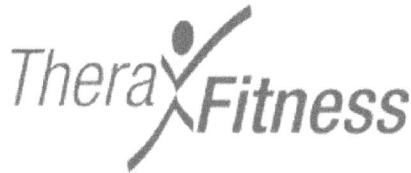

Although originally the name of a specialized exercise class, Thera-Fitness was eventually incorporated for the purpose of promoting programs, products, and physical therapy services.

Today, Thera-Fitness is proud to promote *Aging Safely, Wisely, and Well*, which attempts to simplify the who, what, why, and when of moving and thinking with greater understanding and ease, based on my interest in, and experience with, a wide range of mind-body strategies and techniques. I hope you will revisit it as guidance and inspiration as often as needed, and that you will share it with anyone who wants to transform the ways they move through life.

Here's to aging well . . .

Vicki

https://thera-fitness.com/
vicki@thera-fitness.com

www.ingramcontent.com/pod-product-compliance
Lightning Source LLC
Chambersburg PA
CBHW051323020426

42333CB00032B/3464